Foot & Ankle:

Musculoskeletal Medicine

Produced by:

The Codman Group

A 503C Non-profit committed to enhancing medical education, patient care, and research through the promotion of collaboration, the open exchange of data and content, and the transmission of knowledge across academic networks.

In collaboration with:

www.FootEducation.com

This book is available as a free eBook online at:

http://www.orthopaedia.com/page/Foot-and-Ankle

or at **https://footeducation.com/physician-resources/**

(Follow the link to: *Foot Ebook for Students and Residents*)

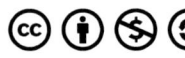

Musculoskeletal Medicine: Foot & Ankle by CODMAN Group is licensed under a Creative Commons Attribution-NonCommercial-ShareAlike 4.0 International License, except where otherwise noted.

CONTENTS

	Series Introduction	iv
	Preface	v
	Peer-Review Note	vi
	List of Contributors	viii

PART I. BACKGROUND

1.	Anatomy of the Foot and Ankle	2
2.	Biomechanics of the Foot and Ankle	18

PART II. CHRONIC FOOT AND ANKLE CONDITIONS

3.	Disorders of the Great Toe	24
4.	Disorders of the Lesser Toes	34
5.	Morton's Neuroma	37
6.	Plantar Fasciitis	41
7.	Tendon Disorders of the Foot and Ankle	46
8.	Achilles Tendon Disorders	52
9.	Arthrosis of the Ankle and Hindfoot	59
10.	Tarsal Tunnel Syndrome	70
11.	Rheumatoid Disorders of the Foot and Ankle	75
12.	Diabetic Foot Disorders	79
13.	Clubfoot	86

PART III. ACUTE FOOT AND ANKLE CONDITIONS

14.	Achilles Tendon Rupture	92
15.	Ankle Sprain	97
16.	Ankle Fractures (Tibia and Fibula)	106
17.	Midfoot Trauma: Lisfranc Injuries	116
18.	Hindfoot Fractures	122
19.	Metatarsal Fractures	133
20.	Stress Fractures of the Foot	140

SERIES INTRODUCTION

Musculoskeletal Medicine is produced by The Codman Group (a 503C IRS-approved public charity) in collaboration with the United States Bone and Joint Initiative and the Community of Musculoskeletal Educators. *Musculoskeletal Medicine* aims to serve as a free, up-to-date, peer-reviewed open educational resource for students and practitioners, thereby improving the welfare of patients.

This Foot & Ankle book was produced from material posted by members of the community on a wiki residing at www.orthopaedicsone.com and from content contained in the website www.FootEducation.com. The content has been edited, peer-reviewed, and then collected into the book you are now reading. A digital version of this book is available online at www.orthopaedia.com or at https://footeducation.com/physician-resources/ (follow the link to Foot Ebook for Student and Residents). We encourage users to visit www.orthopaedicsone.com and improve the content there. The updated wiki pages will be the basis for all subsequent editions – after peer-review, of course.

Please visit http://www.mskmed.org/register/ to join the community and help with this work.

Dan Jacob
President, The Codman Group

Joseph Bernstein, MD, FACS
Christian Veillette, MD, FRCS(C)
Musculoskeletal Medicine Series Editors

PREFACE

Musculoskeletal medicine is typically underrepresented in the standard medical school curriculum: The prevalence of musculoskeletal conditions requiring assessment, diagnosis, and treatment is high, whereas the amount of curricular time devoted to them is low. The discrepancy is likely to widen, as there are a growing number of elderly patients requiring musculoskeletal care without a similar increase in the education about these conditions. Within the broad field of musculoskeletal medicine, where many topics do not get from teachers the attention they deserve, foot and ankle conditions are especially overlooked. The foot is subject to a variety of acute and chronic problems that can be a source of pain and dysfunction to patients. Therefore, it is important that medical students and doctors understand the basics of foot pathophysiology.

This book attempts to explain foot injuries and conditions to medical students and residents in a way that is both engaging and educational. It is the result of a collaboration of a group of committed and experienced orthopaedic foot and ankle surgeons. The chapters have been written to emphasize the key concepts of each condition. The diseases described are those that are most commonly encountered in medical practice. It is our hope that students use this book as a learning tool and also as a reference during their studies at medical school and residency, and throughout their medical careers, regardless of specialty.

Editor: Foot & Ankle Edition, Musculoskeletal Medicine
Stephen Pinney MD MEd FRCS(C)
Chief, Foot and Ankle,
San Francisco Orthopaedic Residency Program
Clinical Lead, Orthopaedic Service Line
St. Mary's Medical Center
San Francisco CA

PEER-REVIEW NOTE

There is a great profusion of medical information available for free on the Internet, and a lot of it is good. Yet even good information may not be completely useful to the reader who may not know if it is trustworthy. By contrast, there is also a lot of information of medical information available for sale that is produced by well known authors and organizations, though not always for free.

Musculoskeletal Medicine aims to be both free and authoritative.

To ensure medical accuracy each chapter was reviewed by an orthopaedic foot and ankle expert who was not involved in the creation of the material. These reviewers were asked to read the chapter with one overriding goal in mind: to detect errors. We are grateful to our chapter editors, listed below:

PEER REVIEWERS

Christopher Arena MD is an Orthopaedic Surgeon affiliated with the Penn State Bone & Joint Institute. Dr. Arena reviewed Achilles Tendon Disorders.

Joseph Bernstein, MD, FACS is Clinical Professor of Orthopaedic Surgery at the University of Pennsylvania.

Jean Brilhault MD is a Foot and Ankle Orthopaedic Surgeon at *Faculté de Médecine de Tours, Université F. Rabelais*. Dr. Brilhault reviewed Achilles Tendon Rupture.

Michael Castro DO is a Foot and Ankle Orthopaedic Surgeon at Summit Orthopedics. Dr. Castro reviewed Ankle Sprains.

Daniel Cuttica MD is a Foot and Ankle Orthopaedic Surgeon at The Orthopaedic Foot and Ankle Center Dr. Cuttica reviewed Diabetic Foot Disorders.

Gwyneth deVries MD FRCSC is a Foot and Ankle Orthopaedic Surgeon at the Horizon Health Network, Fredericton, New Brunswick, Canada. She is an assistant professor at Dalhousie University. Dr. deVries reviewed Metatarsal Fractures.

Christopher DiGiovanni MD is an Associate Professor and Vice Chairman (Academic Affairs) at Harvard Medical School and Chief of Foot and Ankle Surgery at Massachusetts General Hospital & Newton Wellesley Hospital. Dr. DiGiovanni reviewed Morton's Neuroma.

John Early MD is a Foot and Ankle Orthopaedic Surgeon at Texas Orthopaedic Associates. Dr. Early reviewed Plantar Fasciitis.

Daniel Farber MD is a Foot and Ankle Orthopaedic Surgeon and Clinical Assistant Professor at Penn Medicine Orthopedics. Dr. Farber reviewed Stress Fractures of the foot.

Daniel Guss MD is a Foot and Ankle Orthopaedic Surgeon at Massachusetts General Hospital and Assistant Professor at Harvard Medical School. Dr. Guss reviewed Stress Fractures of the foot.

Kamran Hamid MD is an Assistant Professor at Rush University Medical Center. Dr. Hamid reviewed Tarsal tunnel syndrome.

Kenneth Hunt MD is a Foot and Ankle Orthopaedic Surgeon and Associate Professor of Orthopedics and Chief of Foot & Ankle at University of Colorado School of Medicine. Dr. Hunt reviewed Tendinitis of the foot and ankle (non-Achilles).

Paul Juliano MD is a Foot and Ankle Orthopaedic Surgeon, Professor, Vice Chairman, Residency Director at Penn States Hershey Bone and Joint Institute. Dr. Juliano reviewed Achilles Tendon Disorders.

Robert Leland MD is a Foot and Ankle Orthopaedic Surgeon at BoulderCentre for Orthopedics. Dr. Leland reviewed Ankle Fractures.

David Oji MD is a Foot and Ankle Orthopaedic Surgeon and Clinical Assistant Professor at Stanford University School of Medicine. Dr. Oji reviewed Diabetic Foot Disorders.

Mark Perry MD is a Foot and Ankle Specialist at the University of South Alabama Department of Orthopaedics. Dr. Perry reviewed Disorders of the great toe.

Ariel Palanca MD is a Foot and Ankle Orthopaedic Surgeon and Clinical Assistant Professor at Stanford University of Medicine. Dr. Palanca reviewed Disorders of the lesser toes.

Vinod Panchbhavi MD is a Foot and Ankle Orthopaedic Surgeon, Professor, and Chief of Foot and Ankle Services at University of Texas. Dr. Panchbhavi reviewed Clubfoot.

Stephen Pinney MD MEd FRCS(C) is a Foot and Ankle Orthopaedic Surgeon and Clinical Lead for the Orthopaedic Service Line at St. Mary's Medical Center in San Francisco CA. He is also Editor in Chief of FootEducation.com. Dr. Pinney reviewed Anatomy, Biomechanics, Arthrosis of the ankle and hindfoot, and Hindfoot fractures.

Lance Silverman MD is a Foot and Ankle Orthopaedic Surgeon at Silverman Ankle & Foot. Dr. Silverman reviewed Metatarsal Fractures.

David Townshend MBBS FRCS is a Foot and Ankle Orthopaedic Surgeon and Trauma Consultant at Northumbria NHS Healthcare Trust. Dr. Townshend reviewed Plantar Fasciitis.

Anthony Van Bergeyk MD is a Foot and Ankle Orthopaedic Surgeon at Rainier Orthopedic Institute. Dr. Van Bergeyk reviewed Rheumatoid disorders of the foot and ankle.

A NECESSARY DISCLAIMER

Peer-review notwithstanding, this being 21st century America, we must include the following Disclaimer, similar to those found in works produced by well known authors and organizations.

This material was prepared for educational purposes only. We therefore disclaim any and all liability for any damages resulting to any individual which may arise out of the use of the material presented here. We similarly disclaim responsibility for any errors or omissions or for results obtained from the use of information contained here.

This material is not intended to represent the only, nor necessarily best, method or procedure appropriate for the medical situations discussed, but rather is intended to present an approach which may be helpful to others who face similar situations. We cannot can take any responsibility for the consequences following the application of any of the information presented here.

<u>The information provided here cannot substitute for the advice of a medical professional</u>. *Even if a given statement is completely true in the abstract, it may not apply to a given patient.*

The information we offer is provided "as is" and without warranty of any kind.

LIST OF CONTRIBUTORS

CONTRIBUTING EDITORS

We first acknowledge **www.FootEducation.com** and its editors. The content from this website was the starting point for this book.

The final version of this book was produced by editing, refining, and merging raw chapters posted on the OrthopaedicsOne wiki with the *FootEducation* material. The following authors listed below generously contributed to these raw chapters, and even more generously allowed their work to be edited, refined and merged (according to the overall needs of the project). Without a doubt, their efforts were the *sine qua non* of the final product.

Alison Bae, MD	Bridget Ellsworth, MD	Ariel Palanca, MD
Jean Brilhault, MD PhD	Daniel Farber, MD	Vinod Panchbhavi, MD
Joseph Bernstein, MD	Justin Greisberg, MD	Hossein Pakzad, MD
Matthew Buchanan, MD	Daniel Guss, MD	Mark Perry, MD
Michael Castro, DO	MaCalus Hogan, MD	Stephen Pinney, MD
Timothy Charlton, MD	Kenneth Hunt, MD	Meera Ramakrishnan, MD
Marcus Coe, MD	Paul Juliano, MD	Michael Salamon, MD
Daniel Cuttica, DO	Drake LeBrun, MPH	Michael Shereff, MD
Robert Dehne, MD	Robert Leland, MD	Lance Silverman, MD
Sam Dellenbaugh, MD	Eric Malicky, MD	Judy Smith, MD
Gwyneth DeVries, MD	Haley Merrill, MD	Peter Stavrou, MD
Christopher DiGiovanni, MD	Steven Neufeld, MD	Dave Townshend, MBBS
John Early, MD	David Oji, MD	Anthony Van Bergeyk, MD

EDITORIAL ASSISTANCE

We are grateful for the expert editorial help provided by Megan Flinner, www.ManagedByMegan.com

COVER ART

Cover art designed and donated by:

Louis Okafor MD

Department of Orthopaedic Surgery, John Hopkins Hospital

PART I.

BACKGROUND

CHAPTER 1.

ANATOMY OF THE FOOT AND ANKLE

INTRODUCTION

A solid understanding of anatomy is essential to effectively diagnose and treat patients with foot and ankle problems. Anatomy is a road map. Most structures in the foot are fairly superficial and can be easily palpated. Anatomical structures (tendons, bones, joints, etc) tend to hurt exactly where they are injured or inflamed. Therefore a basic understanding of surface anatomy allows the clinician to quickly establish the diagnosis or at least narrow the differential diagnosis. For those conditions that require surgery a detailed understanding of anatomy is critical to ensure that the procedure is performed efficiently and without injuring any important structures. With a good grasp of foot anatomy it readily becomes apparent which surgical approaches can be used to access various areas of the foot and ankle.

There are a variety of anatomical structures that make up the anatomy of the foot and ankle (Figure 1) including bones, joints, ligaments, muscles, tendons, and nerves. These will be reviewed in the sections of this chapter.

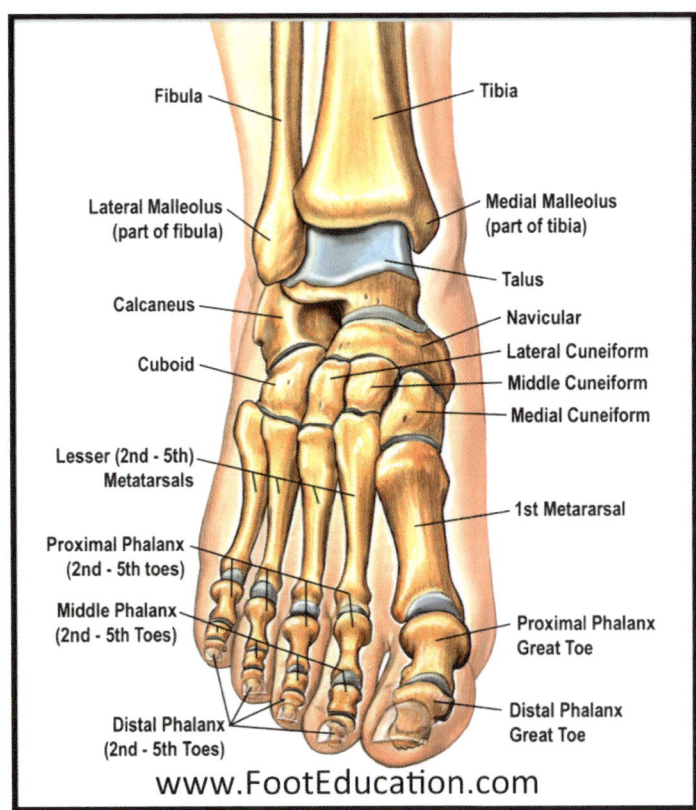

Figure 1: Bones of the Foot and Ankle

Regions of the Foot

The foot is traditionally divided into three regions: the *hindfoot*, the *midfoot*, and the *forefoot* (Figure 2). Additionally, the *lower leg* often refers to the area between the knee and the ankle and this area is critical to the functioning of the foot.

The Hindfoot begins at the ankle joint and stops at the transverse tarsal joint (a combination of the talonavicular and calcaneal-cuboid joints). The bones of the hindfoot are the talus and the calcaneus.

The Midfoot begins at the transverse tarsal joint and ends where the metatarsals begin –at the tarsometatarsal (TMT) joint. While the midfoot has several more joints than the hindfoot, these joints have limited mobility. The five bones of the midfoot comprise the navicular, cuboid, and the three cuneiforms (medial, middle, and lateral).

The Forefoot is composed of the metatarsals, phalanges, and sesamoids. The bones that make up the forefoot are those that are last to leave the ground during walking. There are twenty-one bones in the forefoot: five metatarsals, fourteen phalanges, and two sesamoids. The great toe has only a proximal and distal phalanx, but the four *lesser toes* each have proximal, middle, and distal phalanges, which are much small than those of the great toe. There are two sesamoid bones embedded in the flexor hallucis brevis tendons that sit under the first metatarsal at the level of the great toe joint (1st metatarsophalangeal joint).

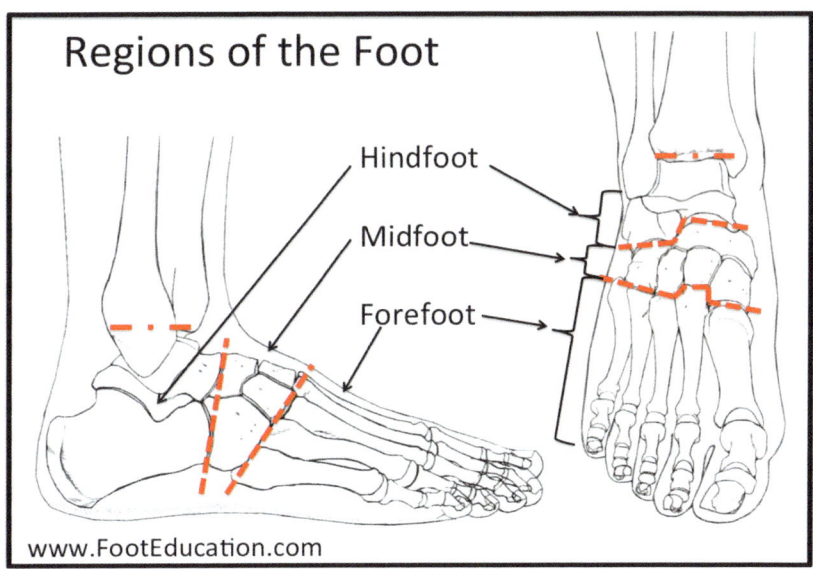

Figure 2: Regions of the Foot

Columns of the Foot

The foot is sometimes described as having two columns (Figure 3). The medial column is more mobile and consists of the talus, navicular, medial cuneiform, 1st metatarsal, and great toe. The lateral column is stiffer and includes the calcaneus, cuboid, and the 4th and 5th metatarsals.

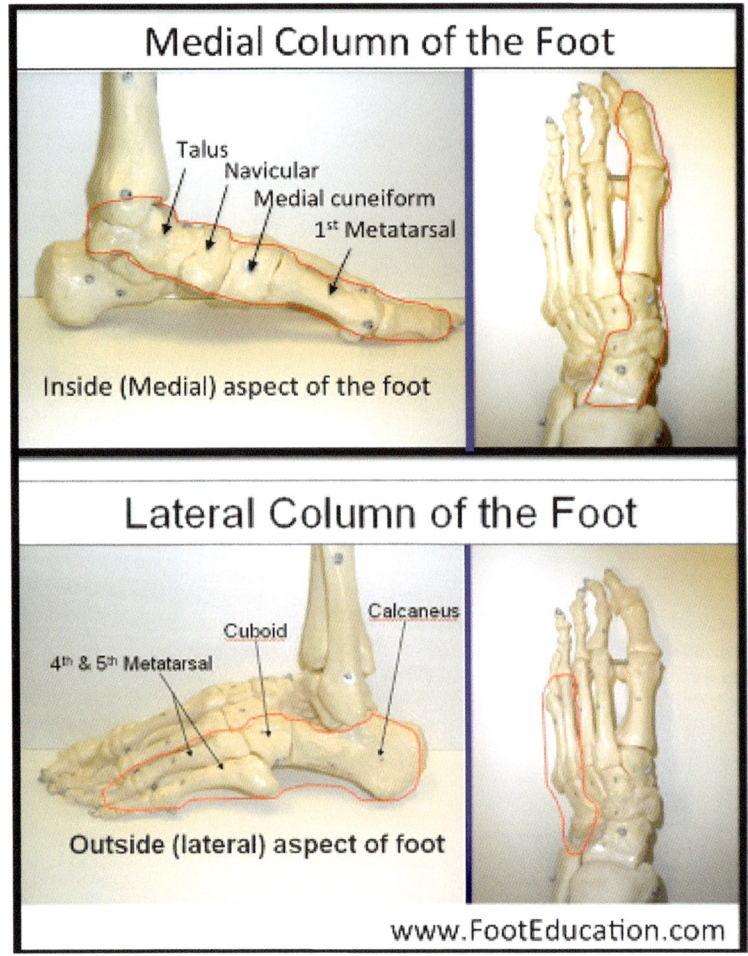

Figure 3: Columns of the Foot

BONES AND JOINTS

The foot is comprised of 28 bones (Figure 1). Where two bones meet a joint is formed –often supported by strong ligaments. It is helpful to think of the joints of the foot based on their mobility (Table 1). A few of the joints are quite mobile and are required for the foot to function normally from a biomechanical point of view. These are often referred to as *essential* joints. There are some joints that move a moderate amount, and there are other joints that are held tightly together with strong ligaments. These non-mobile joints are sometimes referred to as *non-essential* joints. (This may be a poor term in that it incorrectly implies that the joints are not important; they are important. Rather the correct sense is only that movement from these joints is less critical.)

Mobile Joints of the Foot and Ankle (Essential Joints):

Ankle joint (tibiotalar joint)

Subtalar joint

Talonavicular joint (TN joint)

Metatarsophalangeal (MTP) joints

Joints that Move a Moderate Amount:

Calcaneal-cuboid joint

Cuboid-metatarsal joint for the fourth and fifth metatarsal.

Proximal interphalangeal joint (PIP)

Distal interphalageal joint (DIP)

Joints with Minimal Movement (Non-Essential Joints):

Navicular-cuneiform joints

Intercuneiform joints

Tarsometatarsal (TMT) joint "Lisfranc" Joint (a.k.a. midfoot joint)

Table 1: Joint Function in the Foot

Bones of the lower leg and hindfoot: Tibia, Fibula, Talus, Calcaneus.
Joints of the hindfoot: Ankle (Tibiotalar), Subtalar.

Tibia and Fibula (long bones)

The foot is connected to the body where the talus articulates with the tibia and fibula. In a typical foot the tibia is responsible for supporting about 85% of body weight. The fibula accepts the remaining 15%; its main role is to serve as the lateral wall of the ankle mortise (Figure 4). The tibia and fibula are held together by the tibiofibular syndesmosis, a collection of 5 ligaments. The prominence on the medial side of the distal tibia is known as the medial malleolus; the distal aspect of the fibula is known as the lateral malleolus.

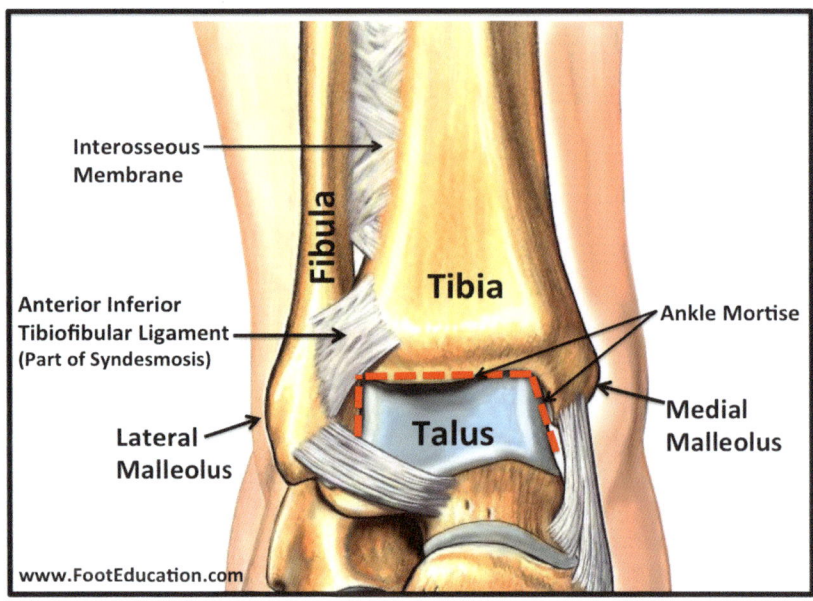

Figure 4: Ankle Joint Anatomy

Talus

The talus is the top (most proximal) bone of the foot. Because it articulates with so many other bones, 70% of the talus is covered with hyaline cartilage (joint cartilage). The talus connects to the *calcaneus* on the underside through the *subtalar joint*, and distally it connects to the navicular through the *talonavicular joint*. These articulations allow the foot to rotate smoothly around the talus. Owing primarily to the fact that no tendons attach to it and that most of its surface is cartilage, the talus has a relatively poor blood supply. The lack of a robust blood supply means that injuries to this bone take greater time to heal than might be the case with other bones—and some injuries will not heal at all.

The talus is generally thought of as having three parts: the body, the head, and the neck (Figure 5). The talar body, which is roughly square in shape and is topped by the dome, connects the talus to the lower leg at the ankle joint. The talar head is adjacent to the *navicular bone* to form the *talonavicular joint*. The talar neck is located between the body and head of the talus. The talar neck is one of the few areas of the talus not covered with cartilage, and is thus the point of entry for the blood vessels supplying the talus.

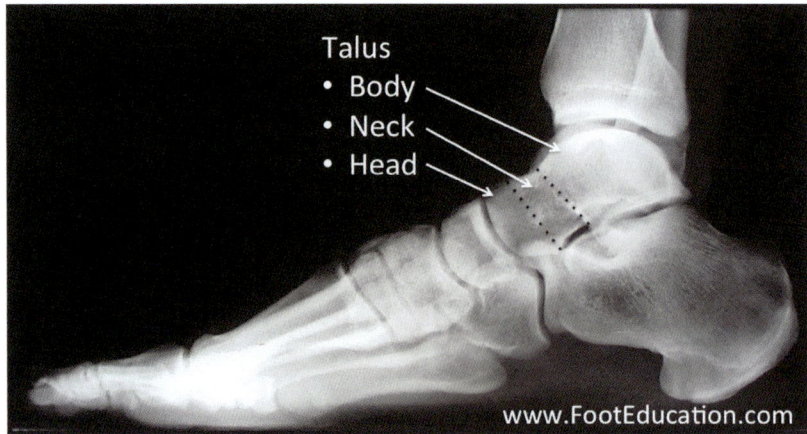

Figure 5: Talus Anatomy

Calcaneus

The calcaneus is commonly known as the heel bone. The calcaneus is the largest bone in the foot, and along with the talus, it makes up the area of the foot known as the hind-foot. There are three protrusions (anterior, middle, and posterior facet) on the superior surface of the calcaneus that allow the talus to sit on top of the calcaneus, forming the *subtalar joint* (Figure 6). The calcaneus also connects to the *cuboid bone* to form the *calcaneal-cuboid joint*.

Subtalar Joint

The talus rests above the calcaneus to form the *subtalar joint* (Figure 6) slightly offset laterally, towards the 5th metatarsal/small toe. This lateral positioning allows greater flexibility in inversion/eversion (tilting). The *subtalar joint* moves in concert with the *talonavicular joint* and the *calcaneocuboid joint*, two joints located near the front of the talus.

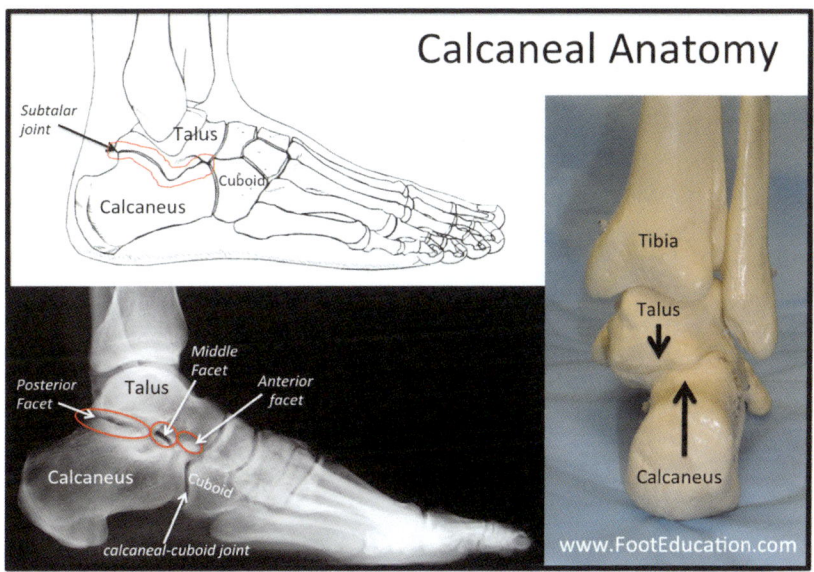

Figure 6: Calcaneal Anatomy

Bones of the midfoot: Cuboid, Navicular, Cuneiform (3).
Joints of the midfoot: talonavicular, calcaneocuboid, intercunneiform, tarsometatarsal (TMT).

Cuboid

The *cuboid bone* is a square-shaped bone on the lateral aspect of the foot. The main joint formed with the cuboid is the *calcaneocuboid joint*, where the distal aspect of the calcaneus articulates with the cuboid.

Navicular

The navicular is distal to the talus and connects with it through the *talonavicular joint*. The distal aspect connects to each of the three *cuneiform bones*. Like the talus, the navicular has a poor blood supply. On its medial side (closest to the middle of the foot) the navicular tuberosity is the main attachment of the *posterior tibial tendon*.

Transverse Tarsal Joint.

The *transverse tarsal joint* is not a true joint, but the combination of the calcaneocuboid and talonavicular joints. When these two joints are aligned in parallel, the foot is flexible yet when their axes are divergent, the foot becomes stiff. The shift from a flexible state to a stiff one allows the foot to serve as a shock absorber and as a rigid level in different phases of gait.

Cuneiforms

There are three cuneiform bones in the foot: the medial, medial (intermediate), and lateral cuneiforms (Figure 7). These bones, along with the strong *plantar and dorsal ligaments* that connect to them, provide a good deal of stability for the foot.

Bones of the forefoot: Metatarsals (5), Phalanges (14), Sesamoid Bones (2)

Metatarsals

Each foot contains five metatarsals, numbered 1-5 medial (great toe) to lateral. The first three metatarsals medially are more rigidly held in place than the lateral two. The metatarsals articulate with the mid-foot at their base, a joint called the *tarsal-metatarsal (TMT) joint*, or *Lisfranc joint*. The TMT joint is made stable not only by strong ligaments connecting these bones, but also because the second metatarsal is recessed into the middle cuneiform in comparison to the others (Figure 7). The metatarsal heads are the main weight bearing surface and the site where the phalanges attached at the *metatarsal-phalangeal (MTP) joint*.

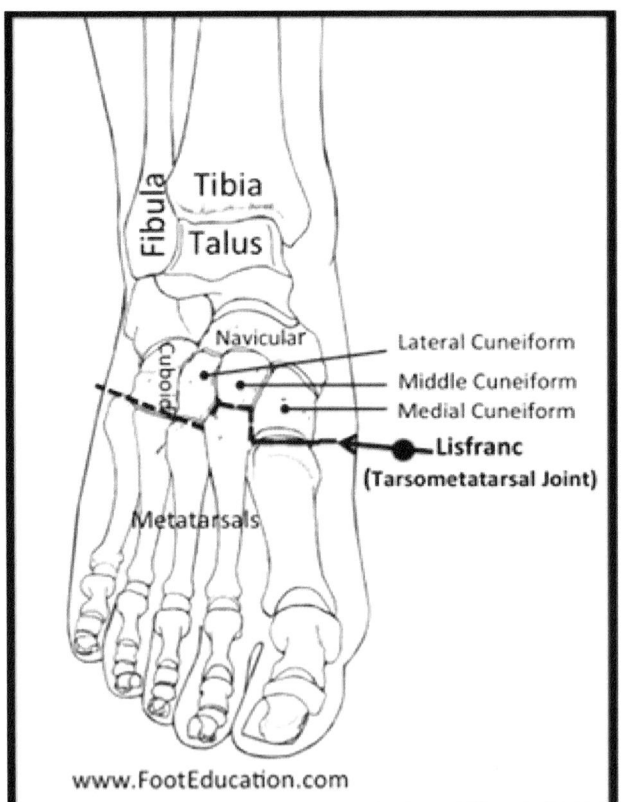

Figure 7: Lisfranc (Tarsometatarsal) Joint

Phalanges

The first toe, also known as the *great toe* or *hallux*, is the only one to have two phalanges; the other *lesser toes* have three. These are known as the proximal phalanx (closest to the ankle) and the distal phalanx (farthest from the ankle). The phalanges form interphalangeal joints between themselves: a *proximal interphalaneal joint* (PIP) and the *distal interphalangeal joint* (DIP) (Figure 8).

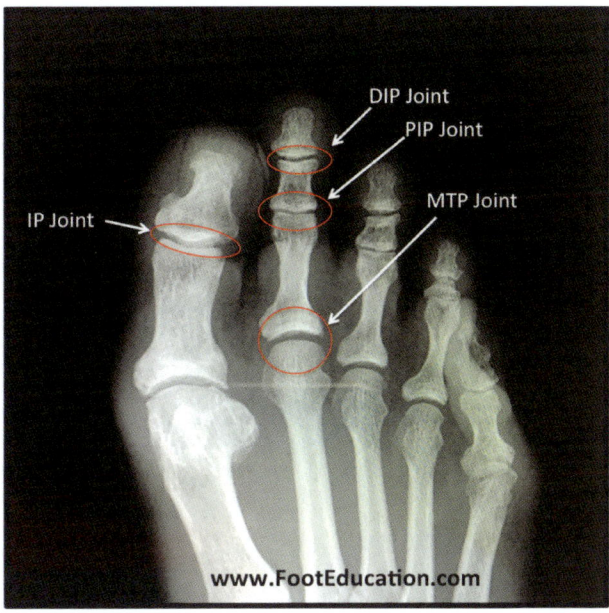

Figure 8: Joints of the Toes

Sesamoid Bones

In the foot, there are two sesamoid bones located directly underneath the first metatarsal head, embedded in the medial (tibial) side and lateral (fibular) aspect of the *flexor hallucis brevis tendon*.

Common Ossicles of the Foot

Some feet contain *accessory ossicles* or *accessory bones* (Figure 9). These extra bones are developmental variants. Over 40 different ossicles of the foot have been reported. The most common accessory bones include:

Os Trigonum: Found at the posterior aspect of the talar body, this ossicle is connected to the talus via a fibrous union that failed to unite (ossify) between the lateral tubercle of the posterior process. An os trigonum is present in about 10% of the population.

Os Naviculare (Os Tibiale Externum or Accessory Navicular): This bone represents a failure to unite the ossification center the navicular tuberosity (where the tibialis posterior tendon inserts) to the main center of the bone. It is present in about 15% of the population.

Os Peroneum: This extra bone is found within the peroneus longus tendon sheath at the point where it wraps around the cuboid. It has been reported in about 20% of patients.

Bipartite Sesamoid: This condition occurs when one of the sesamoids associates with the great toe fails to ossify resulting in two bone segments connected by a fibrous union. It can be mistaken for a sesamoid fracture. Bipartite sesamoids are seen in about 20% of the population with more than 90% of them occurring in the tibial sesamoid.

Os Subfibulare: This extra bone is seen at the type of the fibula. It can be mistaken for an avulsion fracture. It is seen in 1-2% of the population.

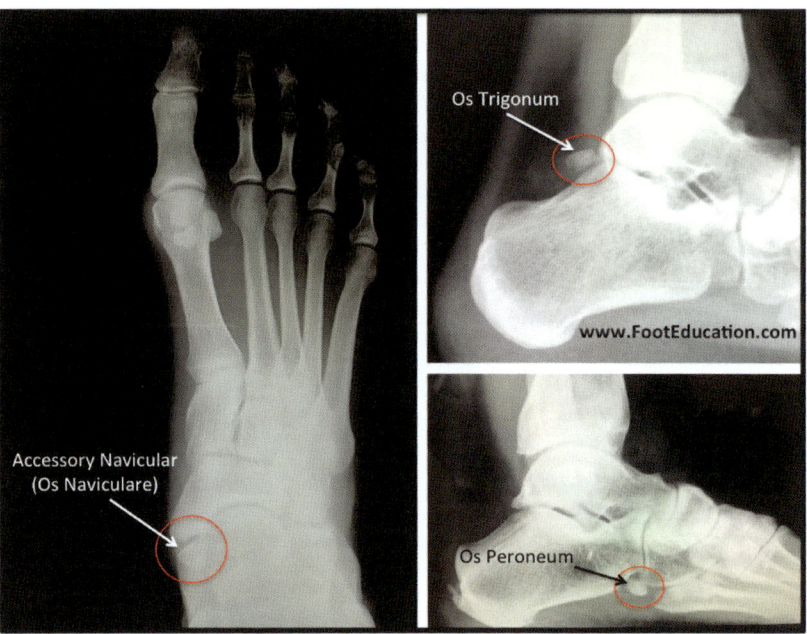

Figure 9: Common Accessory Ossicles of the Foot

LIGAMENTS

The Anterior TaloFibular Ligament (ATFL)

The anterior talofibular ligament (Figure 10) is the most commonly injured ligament when an ankle is sprained. The ATFL runs from the anterior aspect of the distal fibula (lateral malleolus) down and to the outer front portion of the ankle in order to connect to the neck of the talus. It stabilizes the ankle against inversion, especially when the ankle is plantar-flexed.

The CalcaneoFibular Ligament (CFL)

The calcaneofibular ligament (Figure 10) is also on the lateral side of the ankle. It starts at the tip of the fibula and runs along the lateral aspect of the ankle and into the calcaneus. It too resists inversion, but more when the ankle is dorsiflexed.

Posterior TaloFibular Ligament

The posterior talofibular ligament runs from the back lower part of the fibula and into the outer back portion of the calcaneus (Figure 10). This ligament functions to stabilize the ankle joint and subtalar joint.

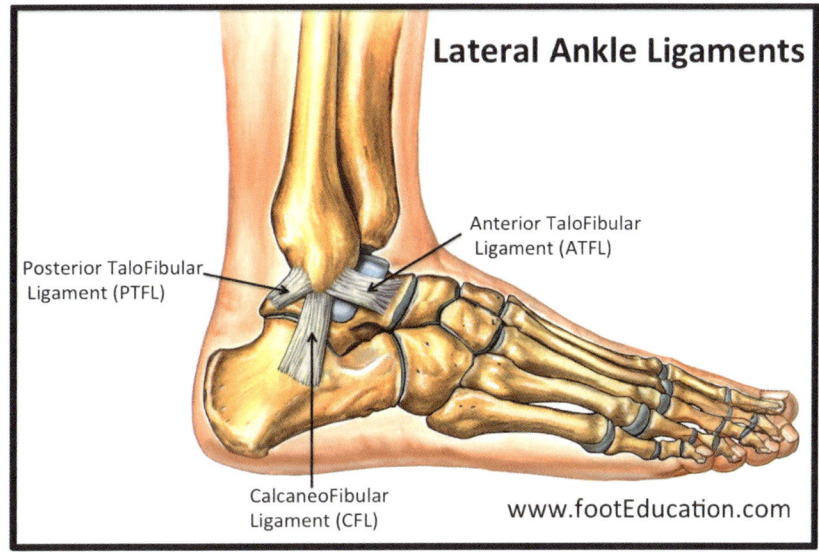

Figure 10: Lateral Ankle Ligaments

The Deltoid Ligament

The deltoid ligament is a fan shaped band of connective tissue on the medial side of the ankle (Figure 11). It runs from the medial malleolus down into the talus and calcaneus. The deeper branch of the ligament is securely fastened in the talus, while the more superficial, broader aspect runs into the calcaneus. This ligament functions to resist eversion.

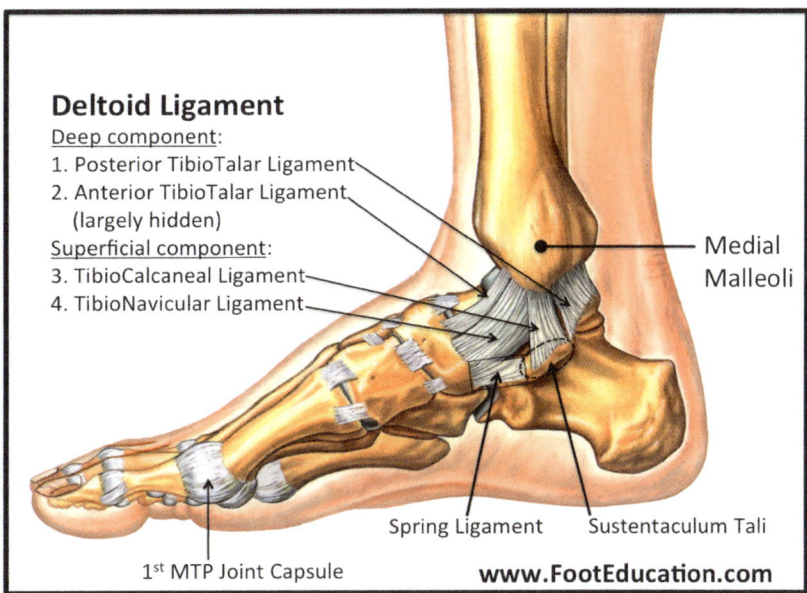

Figure 11: Medial Deltoid Ligament

Spring Ligament

The spring ligament (Figure 11) is a strong ligament that originates on the sustentaculum tali – a bony prominence of the calcaneus on the medial aspect of the hindfoot. The spring ligament inserts into the plantar medial aspect of the navicular and serves to cradle and support the talar head.

Lisfranc Ligaments

The Lisfranc joint complex is a series of ligaments that stabilize the tarsometatarsal joints. These ligaments prevent the joints of the midfoot from moving much, and as such provide considerable stability to the arch of the foot. The plantar ligaments are stronger than those on the dorsal side (Figure 12 & 13). The Lisfranc ligament is a strong band of tissue that connects the medial cuneiform to the base of the second metatarsal.

The Inter-Metatarsal Ligaments

These ligaments run between the metatarsal bones at the base of the toes (Figure 12). They connect the neck region of each metatarsal to the one next to it, and bind them together. This keeps the metatarsals moving in sync. While it is possible to tear these ligaments, it is also possible for them to irritate the digital nerve as it crosses the ligaments creating a Morton's neuroma.

The 1st MTP joint Capsule of the Great Toe

The connective tissue of this ligament takes the form of a capsule (Figure 12). It goes from the medial portion of the first metatarsal head and stretches to the distal phalanx on the same side. This allows this ligament to stabilize the great toe on the medial side. In the situation where a person develops a bunion, this band gets stretched out, and the great toe changes position and becomes angulated outward.

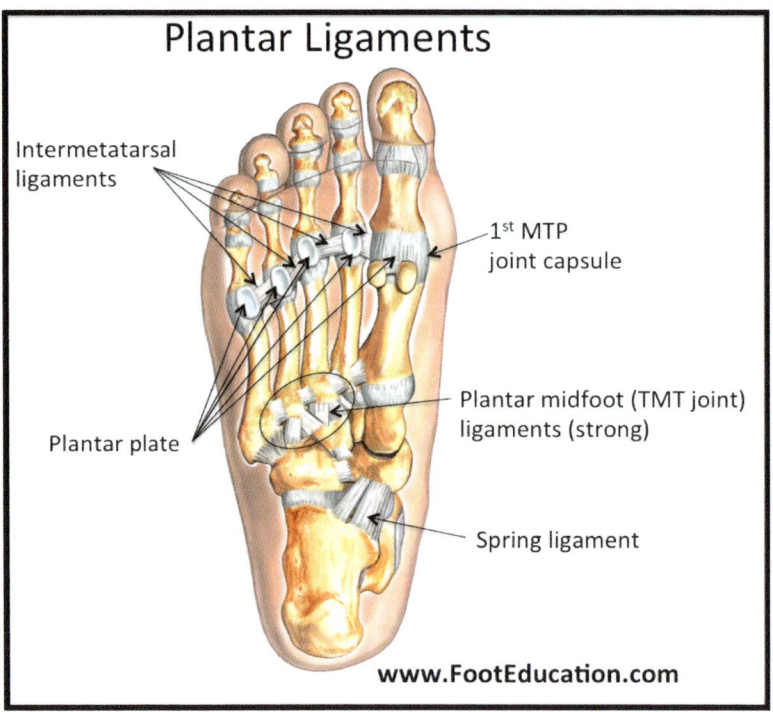

Figure 12: Plantar Ligaments

Anterior Inferior TibioFibular Ligament (AITFL)

The anterior inferior tibiofibular ligament (Figure 4) is positioned on the anterolateral aspect of the ankle joint and serves to helps keep the tibia and fibula together. Injuries to this ligament, so called high ankle sprains, occur when the foot is stuck on the ground while the leg rotates inwards.

The Interosseous Membrane

The interosseous membrane is composed of strong fibrous tissue and runs along the tibia and fibula, and keeps the two bones moving as one unit (Figure 4).

The syndesmosis

The ligament group formed by the AITFL and the interosseous membrane, joined by the posterior inferior tibiofibular ligament, the transverse ligament and the interosseous ligament is known as the *syndesmosis*. The function of the syndesmosis is to hold the tibia and fibula together at the appropriate distance, thereby forming the mortise into which the talus sits

MUSCLES AND TENDONS

There are four muscle compartments in the lower leg (Figure 13) each separated by strong fascia:

1. the superficial posterior compartment;
2. the deep posterior compartment;
3. the anterior compartment and;
4. the lateral compartment

Collectively the muscles in these four compartments are referred to as the *extrinsic* muscles of the foot because they originate above the foot in the leg, but insert within the foot.

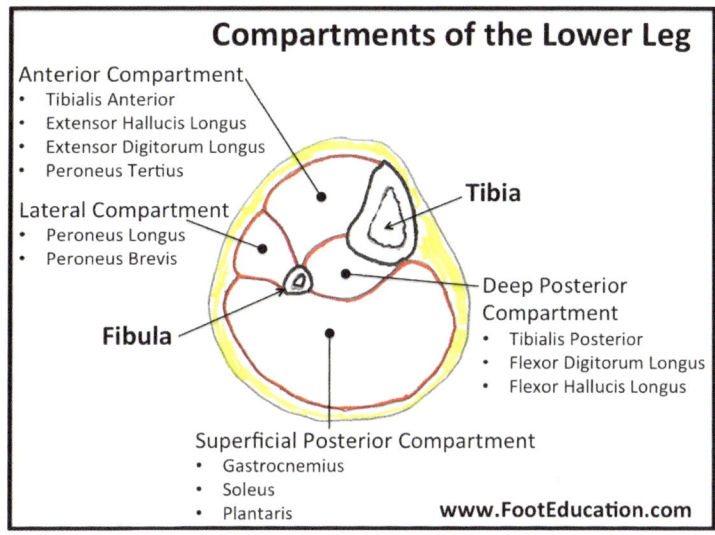

Figure 13: Muscle Compartments of the Lower Leg

Superficial Posterior Compartment

The superficial posterior compartment of the leg holds the two large muscles of the calf, the gastrocnemius and the soleus, which both run along the length of the leg joining to form the Achilles tendon. Both gastrocnemius and soleus muscles are innervated by the tibial nerve. The *gastrocnemius* is the more superficial of the posterior calf muscles. It originates above the knee joint, off the posterior femur, and inserts into the calcaneus. The *soleus* is the deeper of the two muscles of the calf and does not cross the knee. There is a smaller third muscle of the superficial posterior compartment called the *plantaris*. It is very small and not functionally important in most people (but is subject to injury nonetheless).

Deep Posterior Compartment

This muscle compartment is located on the backside of the leg deep to the soleus muscle. There are three muscles in this compartment, the flexor hallucis longus, the flexor digitorum longus, and the tibialis posterior. All three of these muscles cross the ankle and insert on bones of the foot, the hallux, the lessor toes and the navicular, respectively. They are innervated by the tibial nerve.

Anterior Compartment

The anterior compartment is comprised of four muscles that extend (dorsiflex) the foot and ankle (Figure 14). The *Tibialis Anterior, the Extensor Hallucis Longus, the Extensor Digitorum Longus and the Peroneus Tertius*. The deep peroneal nerve innervates all the muscles of the anterior compartment.

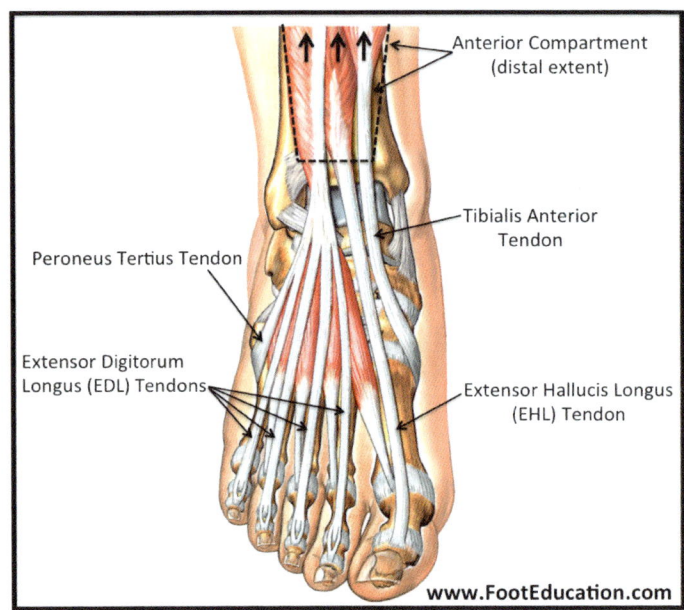

Figure 14: Dorsiflexors of the Foot and Ankle

Lateral Compartment

The last of the muscle compartments of the lower leg is the lateral compartment (Figure 15) is comprised of two muscles, the *peroneus longus* and the *peroneus brevis*. Both cross the ankle, but the peroneus longus wraps underneath the cuboid crossing the plantar aspect of the foot as well, and inserts at the base of the first metatarsal. The peroneus brevis inserts at the base of the fifth metatarsal on the lateral aspect of the foot. These two muscles work together to evert the foot – move it towards the lateral side. The peroneus longus also functions to plantarflex the first metatarsal. Both of these muscles are controlled by the superficial peroneal nerve.

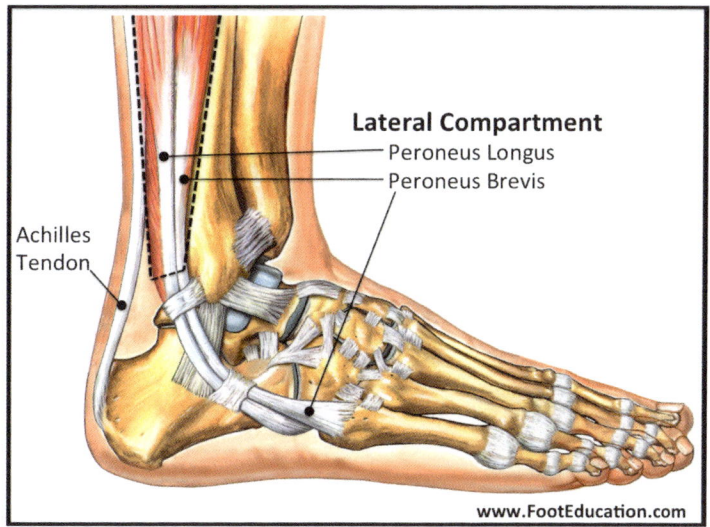

Figure 15: Lateral Compartment Muscles

Muscles within the Foot

There are a large number of smaller muscles deep inside the foot. They help move the toes and stabilize the foot. Collectively they are referred to as the *intrinsic* muscles of the foot because they are entirely contained within the foot. Only two of these muscles are located on the dorsal aspect (top) of the foot: the *extensor hallucis brevis*, and the *extensor digitorum brevis*. They are both innervated by the deep peroneal nerve. Their primary purpose is to help extend the toes. This is in contrast to the *flexor hallucis* brevis and *flexor digitorum brevis*. These muscle tendon units are located deep in the plantar arch and respectively assist in flexing the great toe and the four lesser toes. They are innervated by the medial plantar nerve.

Plantar Fascia

The plantar fascia is not a nerve, tendon or muscle, but rather a strong fibrous tissue (Figure 16). This tissue originates deep within the plantar surface of the calcaneus (heel bone) and covers the distance to the base of each of the five toes. When the foot rolls off the ground during walking, the toes dorsiflex and pull on the plantar fascia. This motion tends to tighten the plantar fascia, and thereby supports the arch of the foot, by maintaining the distance between the calcaneus and the metatarsal heads – a phenomenon known as the *windlass mechanism*. This stiff and relatively impermeable covering helps to protect the muscles of the sole of the foot.

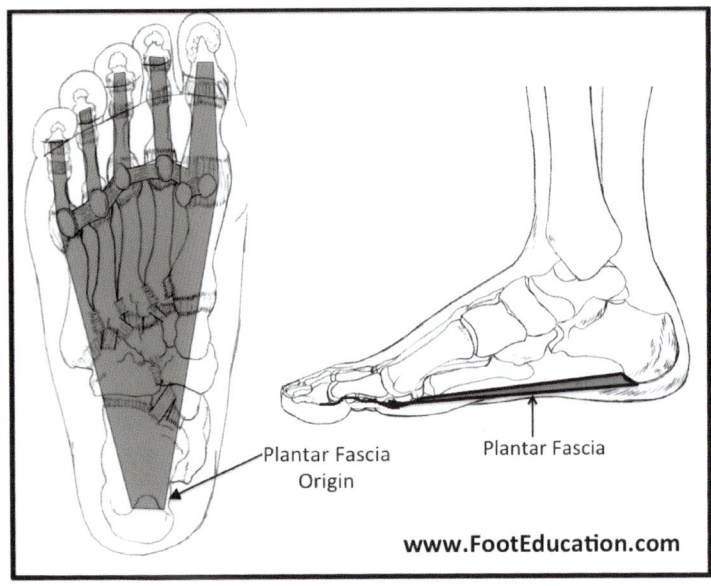

Figure 16: Plantar Fascia

NERVES

Nerves of the Foot

There are five main nerves that run past the ankle into the foot (Figure 17). All five of these are derived from two nerves that originate from the lumbar spine. The *sciatic nerve* branches into four of the five primary nerves of the foot. Two segments of the sciatic nerve branch before the knee joint: the *tibial nerve* and *peroneal nerve*. The tibial nerve gives off a branch called the *sural nerve*. Near the level of the knee the peroneal nerve splits into the *deep peroneal nerve* and the *superficial peroneal nerve*. The fifth nerve of the foot originates from the femoral nerve and is called the *saphenous nerve*.

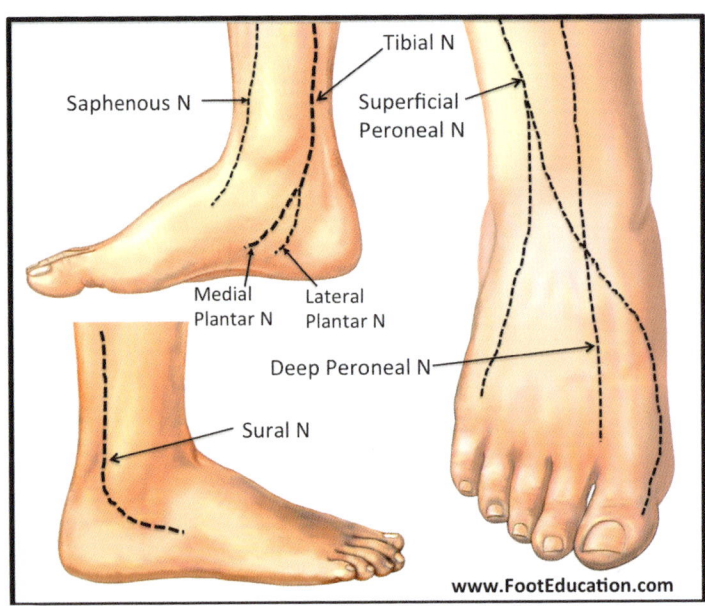

Figure 17: Major Nerves of the Foot and Ankle

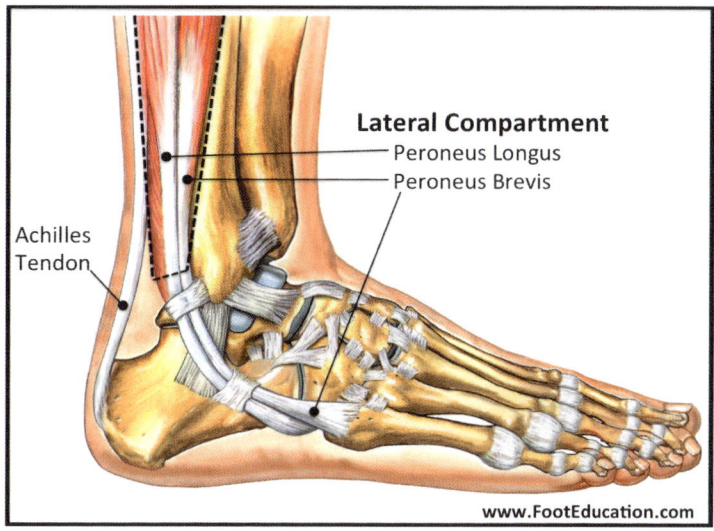

Figure 15: Lateral Compartment Muscles

Muscles within the Foot

There are a large number of smaller muscles deep inside the foot. They help move the toes and stabilize the foot. Collectively they are referred to as the *intrinsic* muscles of the foot because they are entirely contained within the foot. Only two of these muscles are located on the dorsal aspect (top) of the foot: the *extensor hallucis brevis*, and the *extensor digitorum brevis*. They are both innervated by the deep peroneal nerve. Their primary purpose is to help extend the toes. This is in contrast to the *flexor hallucis* brevis and *flexor digitorum brevis*. These muscle tendon units are located deep in the plantar arch and respectively assist in flexing the great toe and the four lesser toes. They are innervated by the medial plantar nerve.

Plantar Fascia

The plantar fascia is not a nerve, tendon or muscle, but rather a strong fibrous tissue (Figure 16). This tissue originates deep within the plantar surface of the calcaneus (heel bone) and covers the distance to the base of each of the five toes. When the foot rolls off the ground during walking, the toes dorsiflex and pull on the plantar fascia. This motion tends to tighten the plantar fascia, and thereby supports the arch of the foot, by maintaining the distance between the calcaneus and the metatarsal heads – a phenomenon known as the *windlass mechanism*. This stiff and relatively impermeable covering helps to protect the muscles of the sole of the foot.

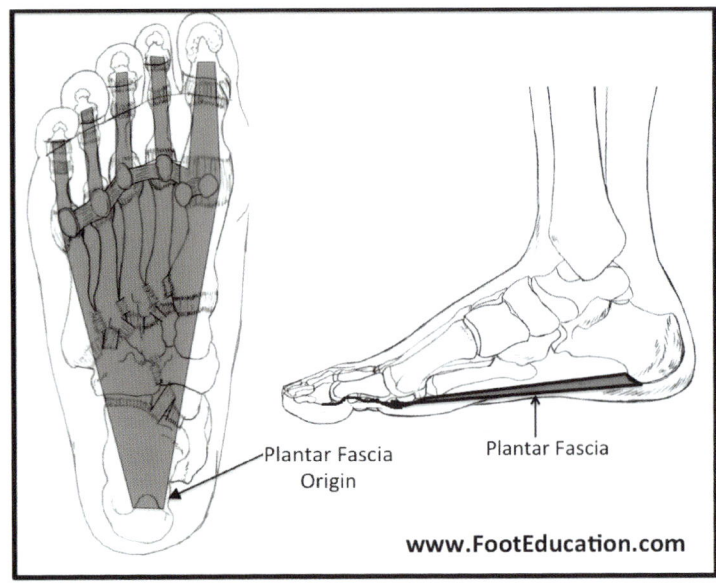

Figure 16: Plantar Fascia

NERVES

Nerves of the Foot

There are five main nerves that run past the ankle into the foot (Figure 17). All five of these are derived from two nerves that originate from the lumbar spine. The *sciatic nerve* branches into four of the five primary nerves of the foot. Two segments of the sciatic nerve branch before the knee joint: the *tibial nerve* and *peroneal nerve*. The tibial nerve gives off a branch called the *sural nerve*. Near the level of the knee the peroneal nerve splits into the *deep peroneal nerve* and the *superficial peroneal nerve*. The fifth nerve of the foot originates from the femoral nerve and is called the *saphenous nerve*.

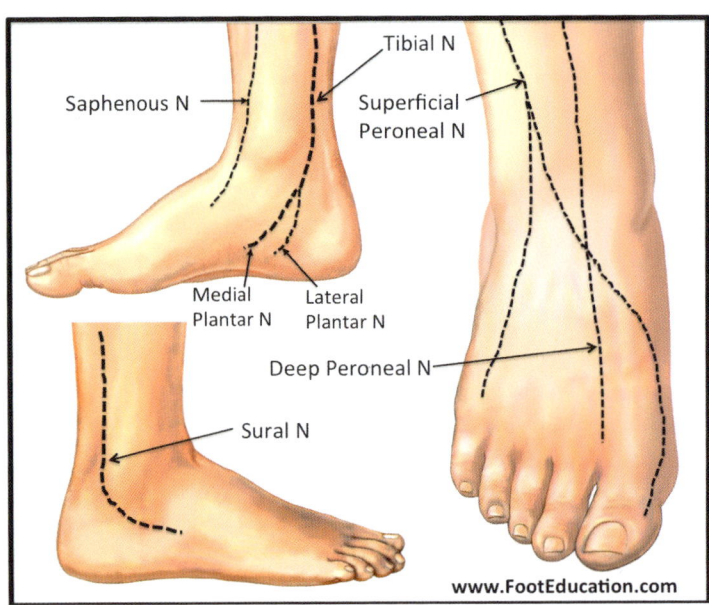

Figure 17: Major Nerves of the Foot and Ankle

The Deep Peroneal Nerve

The deep peroneal nerve is one of two parts of the peroneal nerve (Figure 17). The deep peroneal nerve runs directly under the head of the fibula. It is responsible for controlling the muscles of the anterior compartment of the leg, and continues down the front of the ankle to the dorsal surface of the foot. It is responsible for the sensation in the small area between the first and second toes, an area known as the first web space. If this nerve doesn't function, there will be no sensation in this area. If motor function is lost, it becomes impossible to lift the foot upwards, a symptom known as a "drop foot".

The Superficial Peroneal Nerve

The superficial peroneal nerve is the partner of the deep peroneal nerve (Figure 17). It runs on the lateral side of the leg below the knee under the head of the fibula and innervates the lateral compartment muscles. It runs down over the anterolateral aspect of the ankle and splits into several branches on the dorsal aspect of the foot. The superficial peroneal nerve has both motor and sensory neurons for most of its length, but below the ankle is made entirely of sensory nerves. If motor function of this nerve is lost, it becomes impossible to evert the foot but there is no motor function lost distal to the ankle.

Tibial Nerve

The tibial nerve controls all the muscles behind the tibia and fibula in the back part of the calf (deep and superficial posterior compartment muscles). The tibial nerve continues down into the deep inner part of the ankle and splits into two branches, the *medial plantar nerve* and the *lateral plantar nerve* (Figure 17). These two branches provide sensation to the entire sole of the foot, and innervate all the tiny muscles of the sole of the foot.

Sural Nerve

The fourth nerve of the foot is another branch of the tibial nerve, known as the sural nerve (Figure 17). This nerve runs from slightly below the knee to the lateral aspect of the foot. It becomes a very superficial nerve at the level of the posterolateral ankle and continues distally to provide sensation to the outside of the foot. It has no motor function.

Saphenous Nerve

The fifth and last nerve is the only one to branch off from the femoral nerve (Figure 17). It runs from medial aspect of the knee and runs over the anteromedial aspect of the ankle joint to provide sensation to the inside of the foot.

Although the positions of these nerves are generally as described, there is a certain amount of variability in nerve position. They can be located lower or higher than described. These variations must be considered while performing surgery.

CHAPTER 2.

BIOMECHANICS OF THE FOOT AND ANKLE

INTRODUCTION

A basic understanding of the biomechanics of the foot is essential to diagnose and treat foot and ankle problems. Most foot and ankle problems have a chronic component to them. A rope that is repetitively pulled on will tend to fray over time. Similarly, tendons that get repetitively loaded are at risk for developing tendonitis. Joints that are excessively loaded in an eccentric manner can develop localized cartilage breakdown. This is analogous to a car tire that wears unevenly on one side if it is put on with uneven alignment. A paper clip that is wiggled back and forth over and over again will eventually break and this is analogous to how stress fractures occur. Similarly, ligaments that are repetitively stretched may become loose leading to joint instability. As repetitive forces absorbed by the foot predispose to these conditions understanding the amount and type of force that a foot is subject to, and how these forces vary based on foot-type, weight, and activities is important.

Forces

In technical terms, a force is that which causes mass to accelerate. At a more intuitive level, a force is either a push (compression), a pull (tension) or a twist (torsion). In the foot and ankle, compression is typically applied to bones and joint surfaces and tension applied to ligaments and tendons. Both bones and soft tissues are subject to torsional forces. (In orthopaedics, there is another main category of force, namely shear, in which there is a deformation as parallel internal surfaces slide past one another, which may happen to the cartilage surface. Shear is less commonly encountered in the foot.)

Pathological forces in the foot can be *ground reactive forces* – that is, the force that the ground exerts on the foot during activity – or forces related to *muscle imbalance*. Each muscle tends to have an antagonist: a muscle that pulls in the opposite direction. For example, the antagonists of the posterior calf muscles that plantarflex the foot are the anterior compartment muscles which dorsiflex it. An imbalance between them from, say, a relative weakness in the anterior compartment muscles, will produce an equinus contracture: namely, the foot will be in a "pulled down" position. Similarly, claw toes are another example of a deformity that develops due to relative muscle imbalance – an imbalance between stronger extrinsic muscle and weaker intrinsic muscles pull the inter-phalangeal joints into a deformed position.

Foot Shape

Foot shape also effects how a foot is loaded. In a perfectly neutral foot, forces tend to be distributed evenly. When the foot shape is not neutral, there may be an overload of forces in specific areas. A flatfoot, for example, will tend to have traction forces loading the structures on the medial aspect of the ankle, with compression forces being increased over the lateral aspect to the ankle and hindfoot (Figure 1). A high arched foot (subtle cavus) has the opposite loading pattern: traction forces on the lateral aspect of the ankle and compression forces on the medial ankle. As a result there are a variety of chronic and acute-on-chronic (for example, stress fractures) clinical problems that are caused by the patient's foot shape and subsequent loading pattern.

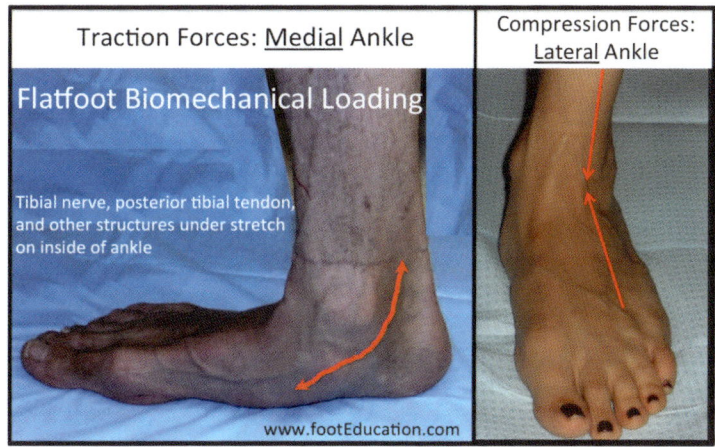

Figure 1: Flatfoot Loading Forces

GAIT

A detailed gait analysis requires sophisticated machinery: high-speed video and force-recording plates on the ground to collect data, and a robust computer program to analyze it. Still, understanding the core elements of gait can improve diagnostic accuracy and treatment recommendations.

There are three areas to focus on when learning about gait:

1) Phases and stages of gait;

2) Movement of major joints (ankle, transverse tarsal joint, etc) during gait; and

3) Activity of specific muscle groups within the phases of gait.

THE FIVE PRIMARY GOALS OF WALKING

Goal 1: The first goal of walking is to move the body forward toward a desired location and at a desired speed.

Goal 2: The second goal of walking is to use the least amount of energy possible to achieve the first goal. During walking, the most energy efficient movement is one in which the body sways side-to-side and bobs up and down as little as possible.

Goal 3: The third goal is to minimize the force applied to painful areas. This can be attained by altering the position of the foot (changing the point of contact with the ground) or altering the gait pattern (that might limit the duration or extent of contact).

Goal 4: The fourth goal for walking is for the foot itself to act as a shock absorber for dispersing the force of the body as it lands.

Goal 5: The fifth goal is for the foot to form a rigid lever toward the end of the phase of gait where the foot is on the ground in order to provide a way to propel the body forward.

THE PHASES OF WALKING

Gait can be divided broadly into a *Stance phase* and *Swing phase* (Figure 2).

Stance phase is the time when the foot is on the ground. It comprises about 60% of the walking cycle. For a brief part of the stance phase, both feet will be on the ground simultaneously

Swing Phase occurs when one foot is on the ground and one in the air. The foot that is in the air is said to be in the *swing phase* of gait.

THE CONSTITUENT STAGES OF THE STANCE PHASES OF WALKING (FOOT ON THE GROUND)

The stance phase has five sub-stages: (Figure 2): *heel strike, early flatfoot, late flatfoot, heel rise,* and *toe off*.

Heel Strike: The *heel strike* phase starts the moment when the heel first touches the ground and lasts until the whole foot is on the ground (*early flatfoot* stage).

Early Flatfoot: The *early flatfoot* stage begins when the whole foot is on the ground and ends when the body's center of gravity passes over top of the foot. The main purpose of the *early flatfoot* stage is to allow the foot to cushion the force of the body weight landing on the foot.

Late Flatfoot: Once the body's center of gravity has passed in front of the neutral position, the *late flatfoot* stage begins. The *late flatfoot* stage of gait ends when the heel lifts off the ground. During the *late flatfoot* phase gait the foot transforms from a flexible shock absorber to a rigid lever that can serve to propel the body forward.

Heel Rise: As the name suggests, the *heel rise* phase begins when the heel begins to leave the ground. Because the foot creates a lever arm when the body's center of gravity is anterior to the point of contact with the ground, the force applied to the foot is at least double body weight. Considering that the average human takes at least 3000 steps per day (an active person commonly takes 10,000 or more steps/day), the foot can easily develop chronic repetitive stress-related foot problems even with normal anatomy.

Toe Off: The *toe off* stage of gait begins as the toes leave the ground. This represents the start of the swing phase.

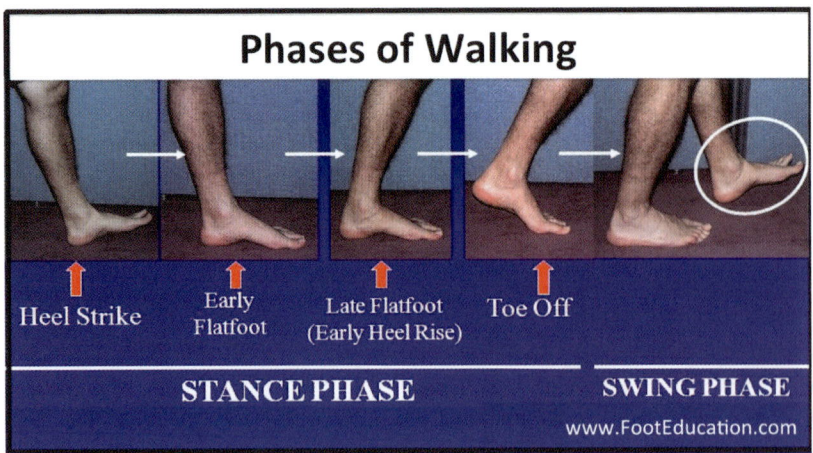

Figure 2: Phases of Walking The phases of late flatfoot and heel rise are depicted in one image in this schematic. The heel rise phase commences the instance the heel leaves the ground.

RUNNING

Walking and running are obviously different in terms of speed, but the formal distinction is that is that during running there is a third phase of gait: the so-called *float phase*. During the float phase, both feet are off the ground. Also, implicitly, because greater speeds require greater energy, the forces applied to the running foot are also greater. Typically, the forces may be four or five times greater than body weight during running and six or seven times greater during sprinting.

FOOT AND ANKLE JOINT MOVEMENT DURING WALKING

With 28 bones in the foot and ankle, there are obviously many distinct points of contact between bones, and technically each of these articulations can be deemed a joint of its own. Nonetheless, it may be reasonable to simplify this and consider only the tibiotalar joint (the "ankle joint" in layman's terms) and the transverse tarsal joint (the combination of the talonavicular and the calcaneocuboid joint).

Ankle (tibiotalar joint) Joint: The tibiotalar joint allows the foot to move up (dorsiflexion) and down (plantarflexion). It is powered by the muscles located in the front of the leg (the anterior muscle compartment) for upward movement, and the muscles located in the back of the leg (the posterior compartment) to pull the foot back down. The main articulating surfaces of this joint are the distal tibia [plafond] and the superior surface of the talus (though of course the lateral wall of the mortise [socket] in which the talus sits is made by the fibula). The hindfoot also contains a subtalar joint, in which the talus articulates with the calcaneus, allowing for a tilt like [inversion and eversion].

Transverse Tarsal Joint: This joint-complex is composed of the talonavicular joint and calcaneal cuboid joint. The transverse tarsal joint is flexible/mobile during the early flatfoot stage, and becomes rigid in the late flatfoot and heel rise phases of the walking cycle. The relative rigidity of this joint corresponds to the two tasks of the foot: the transverse tarsal joint is unlocked when the foot is absorbing shock (*early flatfoot*) and is locked when the foot becomes a lever (*late flatfoot* and *heel rise*). The key to this change is the posterior tibial tendon. This tendon attaches on the navicular, and by pulling on that bone is able to move the axes of the talonavicular and calcaneal cuboid joint, such that the joints are no longer parallel. When these axes are not parallel, the joint locks. This way, when the heel rises off the ground, the calf can channel force into the ground to propel the body forward.

It is important to realize that classic description of locking and unlocking the transverse tarsal joint applies only to an idealized normal foot. A flatfoot often never truly locks to form a completely rigid lever, whereas a high arched foot may never truly unlock and thereby remain relatively stiff throughout the gait cycle.

HOW THE MUSCLES WORK DURING WALKING

Although muscles are reasonably considered in terms of their primary motion they create, it is important to recall that they may be used [and are critically needed] as antagonists to the opposite motion. In simple terms, one may think of the biceps in the upper arm as a muscle that flexes the elbow yet the biceps also works to slow down the extension of the elbow joint when there's a weight in the hand – a so-called eccentric contraction. Indeed, it is during such a motion that the biceps is typically torn.

In the foot and ankle, the anterior compartment muscles (tibialis anterior, extensor hallucis longus and extensor digitorum longus) tend to extend (dorsiflex) the ankle joint, whereas the posterior compartment muscles, via the Achilles tendon, plantar flex it. That said, a critically important function of the anterior compartment muscles to resist the plantar flexion motion produced by gravity and momentum; these muscles gently lower the foot onto the ground during Heel Strike-Early flat foot phases. If these muscles do not work, such as would be the case in someone with a drop foot, the foot will tend to slap onto the ground when it lands.

Similarly, the posterior calf muscles work both in active plantar flexion, as during heel rise and toe off, to propel the body forward, and in resisted dorsiflexion, to decelerate the ankle joint during late flatfoot. The eccentric contraction of the posterior calf muscles during this phase generates an extraordinary mount of internal force and therefore it is during this stage of gait that most ruptures of the Achilles tendon occur.

ABNORMAL GAIT PATTERNS

Antalgic Gait (a "painful walking" limp)

The primary sign of an antalgic gait is the reduced amount of time spent in the stance phase. This is because people do not want to spend any more time than necessary on a foot that is causing them pain. While the stance phase is usually divided equally between the two legs, someone with a painful foot will spend perhaps only 20-30% of their gait cycle in stance. Another related sign of painful gait is a decreased stride length, which results from patients not wanting to push off from their painful foot as powerfully as normal. Taken together, the limping pattern associated with a painful foot is an abbreviated stance phase, coupled with a lengthier swing phase, both in terms of time and distance covered.

High Steppage Gait

A high-steppage gait pattern is seen in patients whose anterior compartment muscles do not function normally (as may be seen in patients with a drop foot from an injury to the common peroneal nerve). Ordinarily, a lack of anterior muscle compartment functioning causes the foot to slap onto the ground during the heel strike phase of walking. Patients respond to this problem by bending (flexing) their knee more than normal during the swing phase of gait (the time when the foot is off the ground). This bent knee tends to keep the foot higher off the ground, and thereby prevents it from slapping.

KEYWORDS

foot biomechanics, gait, ground reactive forces, muscle imbalance forces, compression forces of the foot, tension forces of the foot, phases of gait, stance phase, swing phase, stages of gait, heel strike, early flatfoot, late flatfoot, heel rise, transverse tarsal joint locking, drop foot, antalgic gait, high-steppage gait

PART II.

CHRONIC FOOT AND ANKLE CONDITIONS

CHAPTER 3.

DISORDERS OF THE GREAT TOE

DESCRIPTION

Disorders of the great toe (the hallux, in medical terminology) include degenerative arthritis (hallux rigidus), bunions (hallux valgus), gout, and traumatic conditions (such as sesamoiditis or turf toe).

STRUCTURE AND FUNCTION

There are three joints of the great toe (Figure 1):

1. the first metatarsophalangeal (MTP) joint, namely, the articulation between the metatarsal head and the proximal phalanx;
2. the interphalangeal (IP) joint between the proximal and distal phalanges; and
3. the articulation between the plantar aspect of the metatarsal head and the sesamoids, the two small bones embedded in the flexor hallucis brevis tendon.

It should be noted that a sesamoid bone is one that lives within a tendon; its function is to increase the distance between the tendon and the center of the joint. By so doing, the sesamoid thereby increases the force the tendon applies, by lengthening its so-called 'lever arm'. The patella is probably the best-known sesamoid.

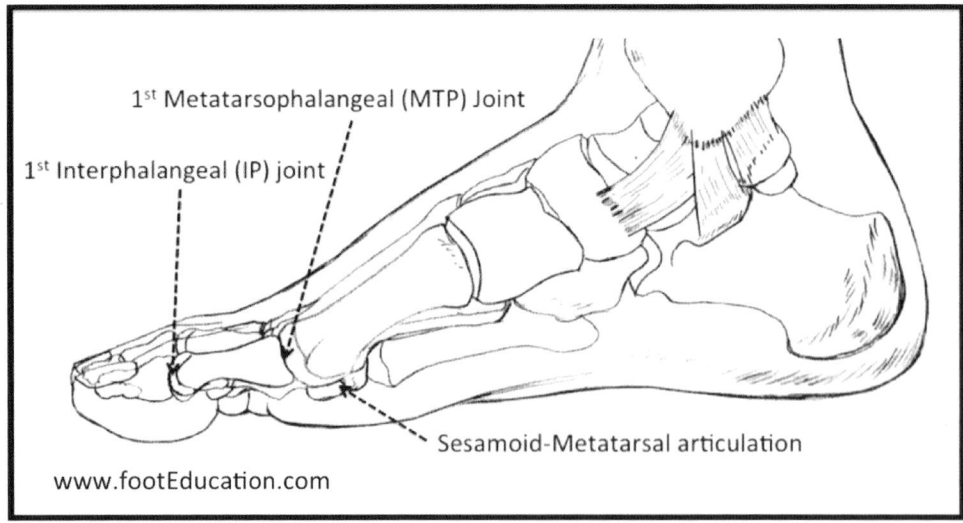

Figure 1: Three Joints of the Great Toe (Hallux)

THE FIRST MTP JOINT

The first MTP joint is a critically important joint. The amount of forces that passes through the first MTP joint and great toe during normal gait varies between individuals depending on foot shape, weight, etc. However, if we consider 6 points of contact in the forefoot (the two sesamoids of the great toe and the 2nd, 3rd, 4th, and 5th metatarsal heads) then we can estimate that the great toe on average absorbs a third (2/6) of the body weight. During athletic activities like jogging and running, these forces can approach two to three times body weight.

Processes that can affect the first MTP joint include overuse; wearing shoes that are too tight or ill-fitting; trauma, autoimmune disease; and deposition of uric acid crystals in the joint (gout).

Hallux Rigidus (arthritis of the big toe)

In hallux rigidus (Figure 2), it is thought that overuse damages the joint surfaces and the nearby soft tissue surrounding the joint. This term is used to describe arthritis of the joint; the name comes to mind because in the MTP joint the osteophytes growing from dorsal aspect of the first MT head impede motion (making the joint rigid) in a way that is not typically seen when osteophytes form near other joints around the body. Of course, the signs and symptoms of the condition include all those of arthritis, not just the rigidity of the joint.

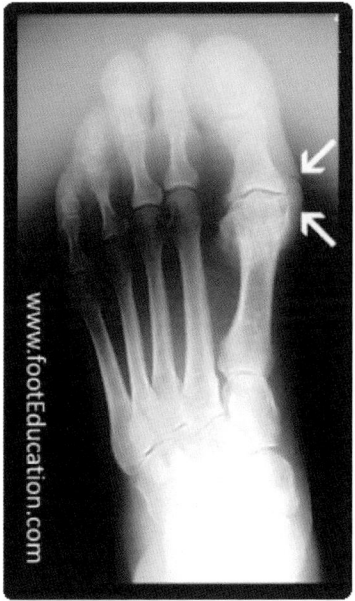

Figure 2: Hallux Rigidus X-Ray

Hallux Valgus (Bunions)

Like hallux rigidus, which is named by one prominent feature, hallux valgus is also designated by one major finding (the valgus deformity of the MTP joint), though it actually comprises several (Figure 3). A valgus deformity is one in which there is deviation at a joint such that the distal bone points away from the midline; in the knee, for example, valgus produces a "knock-knee" configuration. Thus, in hallux valgus there is a lateral deviation of the phalanx (towards the other 4 toes). Beyond that, though, there is also a medial deviation of the first metatarsal along with soft-tissue enlargement of the first metatarsal head. The MTP joint could remain congruent, but eventually can subluxate creating a non-congruent deformity. When there is a loss of congruence, the pull of muscles accentuates the deformity further, and the proximal phalanx progressively moves laterally and the metatarsal medially; the dorsomedial capsule attenuates and the abductor hallucis tendon slides under the metatarsal head. This subluxation of the abductor hallucis tendon pulls the hallux into pronation. In time, there is also lateral subluxation of the sesamoids. In late stages, the extensor hallucis contracts, causing both extension and lateral deviation of the great toe.

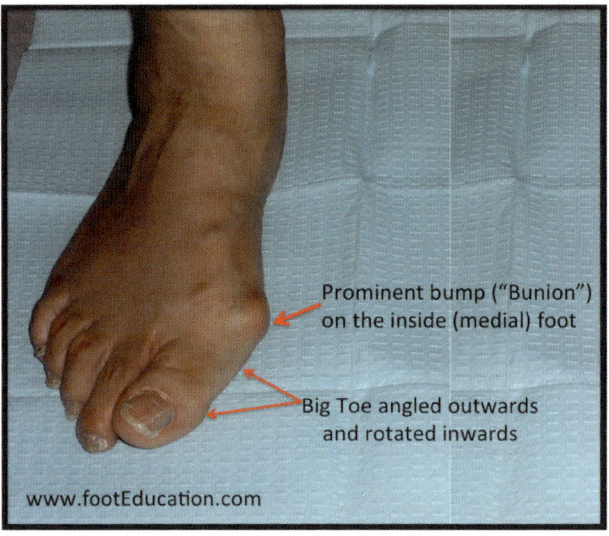

Figure 3: Hallux Valgus/Bunion

Gout (Podagra)

Gout is a painful arthritic condition that can affect any joint, but commonly involves the first MTP joint. Gout occurs when uric acid (urate) crystallizes in the synovial lining of the involved joint. Once in the joint, these crystals induce synovial macrophages to produce inflammatory cytokines such as Interleukin-1 (IL-1). The urate crystals also induce neutrophils to migrate to the joint, increasing the inflammatory process.

Patients with longstanding gout may have masses of urate crystals deposited in soft tissue, cartilage and bone; these are known as "tophi" (singular: tophus). These tophi consist of central deposits of monosodium urate surrounded by fibrous and inflammatory rinds. Small tophi may be asymptomatic; large ones can be painful, even when there is no burst of inflammatory activity.

Turf Toe

Turf toe is an acute injury to the MTP joint that occurs when the great toe is forced upward. This produces an injury to the plantar plate. The classic mechanism is an athlete jamming his or her foot against a hard surface.

Sesamoiditis

Sesamoiditis is a general term for painful symptoms associated with either one or both of the sesamoid bones. The tibial (medial) sesamoid is subject to more force and thus more prone to injury. The mechanism of injury is usually associated with repetitive, excessive loading of this area of the foot, but it can also be due to trauma or forced dorsiflexion. Often patients will have a higher arched foot, causing the sesamoids to be subjected to great force with each step. The resulting pathology may include chronic soft-tissue injury, stress fracture of one of the sesamoids or a sesamoid that never heals (nonunion) after injury, or cartilage damage (arthritis) between the sesamoid and the first metatarsal head.

PATIENT PRESENTATION

Patients with hallux valgus present with a prominent bump on the medial side of the MTP joint. Symptoms range in severity from none at all to severe discomfort aggravated by standing and walking. There is no direct correlation between the size of the bunion and the patient's symptoms – some patients with severe bunion deformities have minimal symptoms, while patients with mild bunion deformities may have significant symptoms. Symptoms are often worsened by shoes with a narrow or stiff toe box.

Physical examination reveals a bony prominence at the medial aspect of the first metatarsal head. The great toe is deviated laterally and often rotated slightly. In mild and moderate bunions, a subluxated MTP joint may be repositioned back to a neutral position (reduced); in more advanced disease, especially if there are arthritic changes in the first MTP joint, the joint cannot be fully reduced. Patients may also have a callus at the base of their second toe under their second metatarsal head in the sole of the forefoot.

Patients with hallux rigidus will typically present with pain, stiffness, and swelling in the first MTP joint (Figure 4). The symptoms are aggravated by repetitive dorsiflexion of the MTP joint (upward movement of the big toe), running, for example. Swelling usually occurs along the top (dorsal) half of the joint, and will frequently be associated with bone spur formation recognized as a "new prominence" by the patient (Figure 6B).

In the early stages of hallux rigidus, there is pain only at ends of the range of motion. In the late stages, there is a loss of motion, especially dorsiflexion, and pain even within the short arc.

Patients may report symptoms from the dorsal prominence (osteophytes). As the condition progresses, patients can attempt to take pressure off the great toe by putting more weight on the outside of the foot as they walk. This may cause metatarsalgia, pain in the forefoot, or in rare instances a Jones fracture of the 5th metatarsal base.

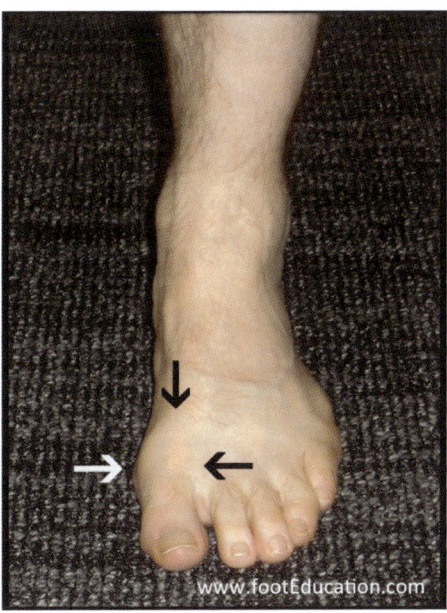

Figure 4: Hallux Rigidus Pain Location

Physical examination will reveal limited and often painful motion in the big toe joint sometimes with crepitus. Prominent osteophytes on the dorsal aspect of the joint are usually visible and palpable. It is very common to see these findings in both feet, although one foot is usually more symptomatic than the other. Tenderness to touch is common dorsal to the swollen MTP joint.

Patients presenting with sesamoiditis will often report a recent increase in repetitive weight-bearing activities that suddenly overload this joint. Rarely is a major acute traumatic event the cause for the problem, although it certainly can be. Pain is typically described as sharp and severe enough to induce a limp. Some patients report that it is especially uncomfortable to walk with barefeet or on hard surfaces. The most common forms of sesamoiditis, by far, presents with a slow, steady onset of patterned pain beneath an otherwise normal looking big toe, which is worse with weight bearing and better with offloading activity. Patients can almost always point to the site of discomfort, which is directly beneath one, or both, of the sesamoids.

It is also common for patients who suffer from sesamoiditis to have high arched feet, due to the higher loads placed on the ball of the foot with this anatomy. Range of motion of the great toe is often normal; marked loss of motion of the big toe, or pain on the top of the great toe is more consistent with a diagnosis of hallux rigidus.

Patients with gout often report a relatively sudden onset of severe symptoms including pain, swelling, and redness. Gout may involve almost any joint in the body, but in 75% of cases, gout affects the first MTP joint (hence the classic name for gout, podagra, which means "seizure" of the foot).

Turf toe injuries result in pain on the plantar surface at the base of the first MTP joint. They usually occur after an acute injury: an athlete will report changing direction suddenly on the playing field, with the great toe forced upwards as the foot is planted on the ground. With enough force, the capsule on the undersurface (plantar aspect) of the great toe will be torn either partially or completely. Patients will complain of pain in the great toe, noticeable swelling, a limp, and an inability to run on the foot. If the capsule is significantly torn the great toe joint may be noted to be unstable.

OBJECTIVE EVIDENCE

Hallux valgus deformity is usually obvious upon physical examination, but it is also easily demonstrated on plain X-ray (Figure 5). A weight-bearing foot series should be obtained to assess forefoot alignment, including the presence of lesser toe deformity, and evaluated for degenerative changes at the IP, MTP, and metatarsal cuneiform (MTC) joints. A weight-bearing anterior-posterior (AP) radiograph assesses hallux valgus angle (HVA), intermetatarsal angle (IMA), MTP joint congruency, and sesamoid position. This evaluation allows for classification and preoperative planning. The lateral radiograph should be assessed for plantar gapping at the 1st MTC joint and dorsal translation of the 1st MT relative to the cuneiform that is indicative of instability.

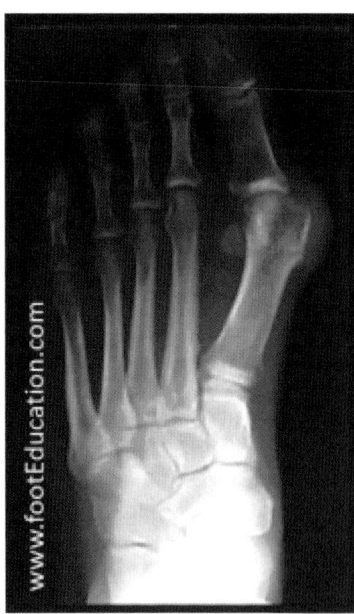

Figure 5: AP X-ray of Hallux Valgus

When hallux rigidus is suspected, weight-bearing foot x-rays should be obtained to demonstrate the presence and extent of MTP joint space narrowing, and identify the location and size of bone spurs. There may be squaring of the metatarsal head on the anterior-posterior (AP) view (Figure 6A). The lateral view will often show a prominent dorsal bone spur (Figure 6B).

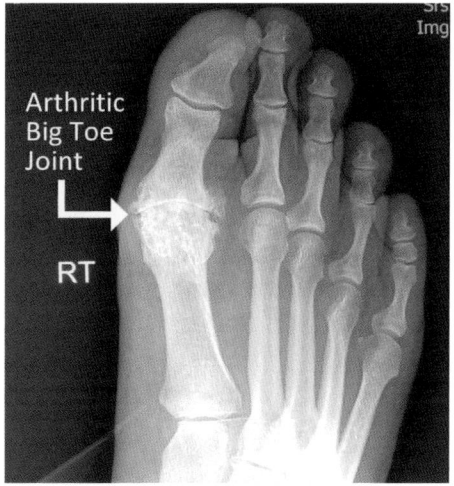

Figure 6A: AP x-ray, hallux rigidus

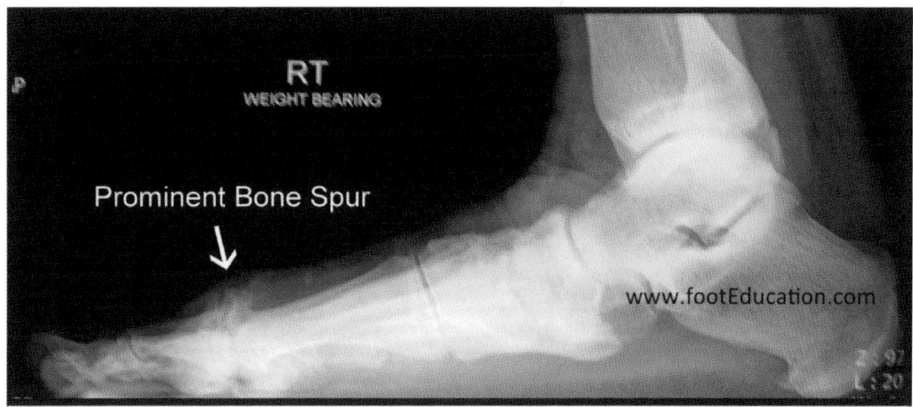

Figure 6B: Lateral x-ray, hallux rigidus

The only definitive way to diagnose an acute gouty attack is to aspirate the joint. Patients with gout will demonstrate synovial fluid leukocytosis (predominantly neutrophils) and the presence of negatively birefringent, needle-shaped crystals viewed using a polarizing microscope. Even with these findings, a simultaneous infection is not definitively excluded. Accordingly, synovial fluid aspirated for gout should always be assessed for infection by Gram stain and culture.

X-rays in turf toe injuries are usually negative, as this injury predominately affects the soft-tissue around the MTP joint. However, plain x-rays should be reviewed to rule out other injuries such as sesamoid fractures and other fractures involving the great toe. A stress x-ray or fluoroscopy may demonstrate excessive movement (instability) of the MTP joint when it is stressed. An MRI will reveal evidence of the soft-tissue (capsular) injury.

When sesamoiditis is suspected, plain x-rays of the foot allow visualization of the two sesamoids and how they sit anatomically beneath the first MTP joint. Fractures, subluxations, dislocations, osteochondrosis, or avascular necrosis affecting the sesamoid(s) can usually be diagnosed on these plain x-rays. It is possible to see fragmentation of the sesamoids that is not pathological: so-called bipartite (two pieces) or multipartite (many pieces) sesamoids. One way to help differentiate a sesamoid fracture from a bipartite sesamoid is by comparison to the contralateral side, as bipartite sesamoids are often bilateral whereas a true fracture is usually not.

When an accurate diagnosis cannot be made and certain possible problems still cannot be ruled out, an MRI scan can usually accurately differentiate between these various pathologies.

EPIDEMIOLOGY

The most common disorder of the great toe is hallux valgus. According to a meta-analysis performed by Nix et al. (PMID:20868524), the prevalence of hallux valgus in patients aged 18-65 is 23% and 35% in patients older than 65 years. In addition to the elderly, hallux valgus is more prevalent in females. There appears to be a hereditary component: a majority of patients have a first-degree family member who also has hallux valgus with the condition.

According to Shereff and Baumhauer, hallux rigidus affects 2.2% of the population 55 years or older (PMID:9655109). It is the second most common condition affecting the big toe after hallux valgus. The condition is often bilateral, and the average age of onset ranges between 12 and 57 years, although it is more common in the older population.

According to Boike et al., sesamoid injuries account for 9% of foot and ankle injuries and 1.2% of running injuries (PMID:21669339). Chronic sesamoid conditions, like sesamoiditis, usually occur in active patients. Sesamoiditis is more prevalent in teens and young adults than older patients.

According to Childs, turf toe prevalence is increasing due to more athletic fields being covered in artificial turf and increased flexibility in the toe-box of athletic shoes (PMID:16900075). Turf toe is seen most often in football players, although athletes participating in basketball, soccer, dancing, tennis, volleyball, and wrestling are at elevated risk. Turf toe is not more prevalent in any one age-group, sex, or ethnicity.

Gout is the most common inflammatory arthritis and its prevalence is on the rise. Putative causes of this rise include the rising prevalence of metabolic syndrome, the aging of the population, and an increase in chronic kidney disease. Gout before the age of 50 is almost exclusively a male disease. At menopause, serum uric acid rises; consequently, gout is present in the older female population as well. Gout is distinctly rare in children, but may occur when genetic mutations affect urate metabolism. The overall prevalence of gout in the US is estimated to be about 3%, but is 10% or greater in older adults.

DIFFERENTIAL DIAGNOSIS

Differential diagnosis for pain at the first MTP joint includes not only bunions (hallux valgus), arthritis (hallux rigidus), gout, and sesamoiditis, but infection, stress fracture, tendon disorders, non-neoplastic soft-tissue masses, and rarely neoplastic soft-tissue and bone neoplasms.

Hallux valgus is fairly easy to diagnose on physical exam. However, it is important to note that asymptomatic hallux valgus can be present along with a second painful condition: a patient with hallux valgus may also suffer from hallux rigidus, sesamoiditis, turf toe, or gout. Therefore, it is important to take a detailed clinical history upon patient presentation even if a hallux valgus deformity is obvious.

While hallux valgus is a fairly obvious diagnosis, sesamoiditis is often a diagnosis of exclusion. It should be considered in active patients who have recently changed their activity level or shoe-wear. Sesamoiditis pain is variable, but often patients will be able to point to the site of pain as being underneath one or both sesamoid bones. The differential diagnosis for this type of pain includes fractures, subluxations, dislocations, osteochondrosis, or avascular necrosis. These can usually be distinguished by plain x-ray.

Hallux rigidus, like sesamoiditis, is also characterized by pain with dorsiflexion and shifting weight laterally during ambulation to avoid toe-off. However, hallux rigidus usually develops over a longer period of time than sesamoiditis. Furthermore, the dorsal aspect of the first MTP joint is normally tender upon palpation in patients with hallux rigidus, while the plantar aspect is tender in patients with sesamoid disorders. Additionally, these two disorders can be differentiated using imaging, as hallux rigidus is characterized by osteophytes on the dorsal aspect of the MTP joint with or without joint space narrowing, while these features are absent in sesamoid disorders. Hallux rigidus must also be differentiated from gout.

Differential diagnosis of acute gout depends on the patient history, physical examination, and laboratory testing. The most important alternative diagnosis to consider, particularly in monoarticular attacks, is septic joint because infection can rapidly and permanently damage joints. Other crystals, particularly calcium crystals, can cause attacks mimicking gout. Gout can also mimic virtually any inflammatory arthritis, depending on the pattern of presentation. For example, rheumatoid arthritis may need to be considered if the gouty attack is polyarticular and involves the hands.

When an athlete presents with an acute injury of the first MTP joint following forced hyper-extension of the hallux, the diagnosis is almost certainly turf toe. However, turf toe is a broad category that encompasses different severities of capsular injury, from attenuation of the capsule (plantar plate) to a complete tear. Plain x-rays should be reviewed to rule out other injuries such as sesamoid fractures and other fractures involving the great toe.

RED FLAGS

Imaging studies should be performed in most cases of first MTP joint pain, especially with recalcitrant pain following conservative treatment, in facilitate an accurate diagnosis and plan future treatments accordingly.

A single gout attack is extremely painful but usually self-limited. A missed diagnosis at that time will be of little long-term consequence. However, a missed diagnosis of an infected joint can be catastrophic; and because gout and infection are often clinically indistinguishable, diagnostic joint aspiration should almost always be performed.

TREATMENT OPTIONS AND OUTCOMES

Non-operative treatment of most causes of great toe pain is usually successful. Conservative treatment strategies include:

1. Activity modification: limiting the extent of weight-bearing activities such as standing and walking in the short and intermediate term decreases the repetitive load and subsequent irritation to the joint and surrounding tissues.
2. Shoe wear modification: Stiff-soles shoes with a soft insert and a wide accommodative toe box can be very helpful in alleviating repetitive irritation and pain from most common great toe conditions.
3. Anti-inflammatory medication (NSAIDs): Short-term use of anti-inflammatory medications can help improve symptoms.
4. Steroid injection: Corticosteroid injections of the 1st MTP joint may be beneficial in recalcitrant cases of hallux rigidus, gout and other conditions where there is marked painful swelling and inflammation of the great toe joint.

The vast majority of great toe problems can be managed non-operatively. The primary indication for operative intervention should be pain that is not relieved by appropriate non-operative management.

Surgical treatment of Bunions (hallux valgus)

Operative treatment for hallux valgus is often requested for cosmetic reasons, but sharing with patients the prolonged recovery time and risks of complications are conveyed, may dissuade them. There are many different surgical treatments for hallux valgus described in the orthopaedic literature. The type of procedure chosen depends on the severity of hallux valgus, co-morbid conditions, and the preference of the surgeon. Some of the common procedures include removal of the medial eminence; a distal metatarsal osteotomy (chevron) with tightening of the medial capsule; a proximal metatarsal osteotomy; great toe fusion (1st MTP joint arthrodesis); or resection arthroplasty (removal of the proximal aspect of the proximal phalanx). Often, up to 12 months are required before maximal recovery is achieved. Post-surgical complications are not uncommon and may include: wound healing problems, infection, nonunion, local nerve injury, deep venous thrombosis (DVT), and pulmonary embolism (PE). Additionally, the deformity may recur, or a new deformity may form at the osteotomy, requiring an additional surgery.

Surgical treatment of Great Toe Arthritis (hallux rigidus)

Operative treatment for hallux rigidus may be indicated when non-operative treatments fail. Surgical treatment of hallux rigidus includes: a 1st MTP joint dorsal cheilectomy (bone spur removal); fusion of the first MTP joint, and first MTP joint arthroplasty or hemiarthroplasty (first MTP joint replacement or partial joint replacement). The dorsal cheilectomy procedure is effective only for patients who have arthritis involving just the dorsal aspect of the first MTP joint; it is not indicated in patients with arthritis involving the entire joint. Recurrence of pain is a not-infrequent complication of cheilectomy. If this is found, the other two surgical options should be considered. Fusion of the great toe joint offers predictable pain relief. One of the defining features of severe hallux rigidus is a loss of 1st MTP joint motion so from a functional point of view loss of joint motion following a fusion is often not a major issue. Joint replacements of the 1st MTP can provide good short and intermediate term pain relief and function. However, eventual failure of the implant can make revision surgery very challenging.

Surgical Treatment of Sesamoiditis

Recalcitrant sesamoiditis that does not improve with 6 months of non-operative treatment can be considered for operative removal of the sesamoids, though most patients recover before that deadline. Excising only the painful sesamoid bone may lead to destabilization of the joint with the development of a subsequent hallux varus or valgus deformity depending on which sesamoid is removed.

Surgical treatment of Turf Toe Injuries

In turf toe injuries where there is complete tearing of the plantar soft-tissues of the great toe (ex. great toe dislocation) surgical repair is indicated. Additionally, turf toe injures resulting in partial tearing of the plantar capsule that do not adequately recover with conservative treatment may benefit from debridement (e.g., cleaning out cartilage debris) and repair of the torn plantar capsule. Recovery can be prolonged: 6 weeks of limited weight-bearing to allow the capsular repair to heal; 6 weeks of controlled rehabilitation in a boot or stiff soled shoe; and 6 or more weeks of sports-specific exercises. It is also not uncommon to have some residual symptoms even after a seemingly successful surgery. Unfortunately, for some athletes, a severe turf toe injury may be a career ending injury.

Treatment of Gout

Treatment of acute gout focuses on suppressing inflammation. Three classes of agents are used: non-steroidal anti-inflammatory drugs, glucocorticoids, and colchicine. All are effective; the choice of agent depends on which will be best tolerated in the individual patient. Intra-articular glucocorticoid injections are effective but should be avoided until infection is definitively excluded. Changing the dose of urate-lowering drugs during an acute attack should generally be avoided because acute urate shifts may worsen the attacks.

For patients with established gout (two or more attacks/year) who are between attacks, urate-lowering should be initiated to reduce the urate burden and the risk of both attacks and tophi. First-line agents include allopurinol and febuxostat, which block urate production by inhibiting the synthesis enzyme xanthine oxidase. In contrast to targeting urate production, probenecid promotes urate excretion from the kidneys. All patients starting urate-lowering therapy must receive anti-inflammatory prophylaxis (usually colchicine) for 6 or more months, since urate lowering transiently increases the risk of gouty attack. The goal is to drive the serum urate level to <6.0 mgs/dL (lower to resolve tophi).

RISK FACTORS AND PREVENTION

Risk factors for hallux rigidus include an elevated first metatarsal and/or a supinated forefoot leading to dorsal jamming at the 1st MTP joint. These risk factors are not really subject to modification. Wearing good comfort shoes (e.g., the correct size, soft uppers, and a stiff sole that limits motion of the first MTP joint) and maintaining a healthy weight, may help in patients who are predisposed to develop hallux rigidus.

Patients with hallux valgus often have a positive family history. The majority of patients with hallux valgus have a first-degree relative who has had a bunion, flatfoot deformity, or significant clawing of their lesser toes. Wearing tight or ill-fitting shoes may contribute to symptoms related to the hallux valgus deformity, but the evidence on causality is not conclusive.

The main risk factor for disorders of the sesamoid is having a higher arched foot. People with high arches that may be predisposed to sesamoiditis may be able to prevent this by wearing shoe inserts that reduce the stress on the sesamoids.

According to Childs, risk factors for turf toe include participating in athletics on artificial turf fields, playing certain sports that predispose to the injury (football, soccer, basketball, wrestling, dancing, tennis, and volleyball), foot pronation, increased toe box flexibility, flat feet, hallux degenerative joint disease, and prior first MTP joint injury (PMID:16900075). Therefore, turf toe injuries may be reduced by wearing shoes with a stiffer sole and limiting the amount of play on artificial turf fields.

Multiple risk factors promote hyperuricemia and subsequently gout. Diets rich in purines, or high in alcohol or fructose (promoting purine turnover and urate synthesis), can raise serum uric acid (sUA). Diseases of high cell turnover such as leukemia and lymphoma also promote hyperuricemia (secondary overproduction). Diuretics and certain other drugs can inhibit renal urate excretion and promote hyperuricemia. Obesity is also associated with hyperuricemia, but the relative contributions of diet versus adiposity are unclear. Nonetheless, weight loss reduces sUA and is advisable in overweight gout patients.

MISCELLANY

Turf toe was so named as the injury became more common with the increasing popularity of artificial turf over natural grass.

Sesamoids are so named because they are thought to resemble sesame seeds.

KEY TERMS

Hallux valgus, Bunion, Hallux rigidus, Great toe arthritis, Gout, Sesamoiditis, Turf toe, Podagra

SKILLS

Perform a thorough musculoskeletal history and physical. Identify pathology on radiographs.

CHAPTER 4.

DISORDERS OF THE LESSER TOES

DESCRIPTION

An imbalance between the extrinsic and intrinsic muscles of the foot can produce deformities of the lesser toes. These deformities are classified by how the separate toe joints are affected. Hammertoe deformities are characterized by flexion of the proximal interphalangeal (PIP) joint and extension of the metatarsal-phalangeal (MTP) joint resulting in a prominent bump at the PIP joint. Claw toe deformities also have PIP flexion and MTP extension but additionally have flexion of the distal interphalangeal (DIP) joint which produces "clawing." Only the DIP joint is affected in mallet toe deformities, so the MTP and PIP joints are naturally extended but the DIP joint is flexed.

STRUCTURE AND FUNCTION

The lesser toes have three phalanges. The proximal phalanx articulates proximally with the metatarsal (at the MTP joint) and distally with the middle phalanx (at the PIP) joint; the middle phalanx's articulation with the distal phalanx is called the DIP joint.

The extensor digitorum longus (EDL), an extrinsic muscle, is the primarily extender of the MTP joint. The extensor digitorum brevis (EDB), an intrinsic muscle, extends the PIP and DIP joints.

The flexor digitorum longus (FDL), another extrinsic muscle, flexes all three joints of the lesser toes, but the DIP joint especially. The flexor digitorum brevis (FDB) tendon (intrinsic) primarily flexes the PIP joint. The lumbricals originate from the metatarsals and flex the MTP joint and extend the PIP and DIP joints.

All of the toe joints have a fibrocartilaginous plantar plate, which passively resist extension as well.

Claw toes are caused by an imbalance between the extrinsic and the intrinsic muscles in the foot, causing flexion at the PIP (proximal interphalangeal) joint and extension at the MTP (metatarsal phalangeal) joint. The PIP joints become prominent and can be irritated by shoes, leading to painful calluses on the dorsal aspect of the toes (Figure 1).

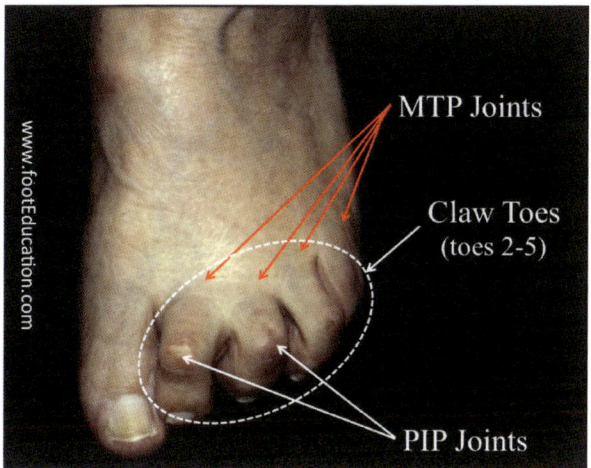

Figure 1: Claw toes. The second toe is usually the most pronounced deformity, but all four lesser toes demonstrate clawing.

Typically, when only a single toe is clawed, trauma or arthritis in the cause. More commonly all four lesser toes are involved and hereditary muscle imbalance (extrinsics > instrinsics) or nerve damage (neuropathy) is the cause.

Hammer toes are usually caused by shoes that force the toe to bend; they are also seen in patients with bunions.

A mallet toe, (i.e. isolated flexion of the DIP joint), may be caused by shoe pressure (causing, eventually, attenuation of the extensor tendon); a tight flexor digitorum longus can also be the cause.

PATIENT PRESENTATION

A patient with a deformity of the lesser toes is very likely an older female presenting with pain on the top of the toes (as they rub against the shoes). There also can be pain on the tip of the toes as they jam into the soles of the shoes. With a long-standing deformity, there can be pain at the base of the toes along with corns or calluses of the skin from repeated friction.

OBJECTIVE EVIDENCE

The deformity is usually obvious, and x-rays confirm what is seen clinically. On physical exam, each joint should be assessed as to whether it can be passively corrected; that is whether the deformities are flexible or rigid (as this guides treatment). It is also important to assess the toes in various positions of ankle flexion/extension, so the effect of any extrinsic muscle tightness can be demonstrated (i.e., tightness of the extrinsic flexors would be worsened with ankle dorsiflexion). Also, because toe deformities are seen as a manifestation of neurological disease, a detailed assessment of strength and sensation is needed.

EPIDEMIOLOGY

Claw toes can be congenital or acquired, and so are seen throughout all ages, though more common with increasing age (the 7th and 8th decades). Women are affected four to five times more than men.

DIFFERENTIAL DIAGNOSIS

Underlying associated conditions include:

- diabetes, with peripheral neuropathy
- rheumatoid arthritis
- primary neuromuscular disease (poliomyelitis, Freidrich's ataxia, myelopathy, multiple sclerosis or Charcot Marie Tooth Disease
- other foot deformities such as bunions, flat feet, or pes cavus deformity (highly arched feet)

RED FLAGS

All lesser toe deformities are red flag findings, suggesting the presence of a complication of diabetes or a neurological disorder. Close evaluation of the whole patient is essential.

TREATMENT OPTIONS AND OUTCOMES

Non-operative

Most deformities can be treated by applying pads to the areas of prominence or using a shoe with a wide-toe box to accommodate the deformity and alleviate pain. Some patients may need an orthotic to create cushioning over the toe region. Trimming painful calluses can relieve symptoms, but without addressing the deformity, they may recur.

Operative

Surgery is considered only in deformities that cannot be corrected non-operatively.

Claw and hammer toes with a flexible deformity may be treated with a flexor and/or extensor tenotomy or a flexor to extensor tendon transfer with a capsular and extensor tendon release. If there is a fixed deformity at the MTP joint, a capsular release and extensor tendon lengthening may suffice. In some patients a metatarsal shortening osteotomy may be needed, especially if the patient has metatarsalgia or tenderness. A fixed PIP deformity is treated with resection arthroplasty or Interphalangeal fusion.

A mallet toe with a flexible deformity can be treated with a percutaneous flexor tenotomy; a rigid deformity requires either a resection arthroplasty of the distal aspect of the middle phalanx or DIP fusion.

Note that the recovery period for any toe surgery is prolonged. It is not uncommon to note swelling and stiffness in the toes even 6 months post-surgery.

Foot surgery, in general, is more susceptible to wound complications and infection; toe deformity surgery, in particular, can be complicated by recurrence of the deformity.

SKILLS

Claw/hammer/mallet toes are typically present in older age or as an indication of an underlying neurological disorder – asking the right questions to the patient and ordering the necessary exams to identify the cause is important.

KEY TERMS

claw toe, hammer toe, mallet toe, lesser toe deformity, metatarsalgia, corns, muscular imbalance

CHAPTER 5.

MORTON'S NEUROMA

DESCRIPTION

Morton's neuroma (also known as an intermetatarsal or interdigital neuroma) is a common cause of forefoot pain. It presents as a sharp, burning sensation in the affected web-space, which often radiates proximally or distally between the adjacent toes; most typically, it is found in the 3-4 or 2-3 intermetatarsal space, which can manifest as pain, burning, and/or numbness between the 3rd and 4th or 2nd and 3rd toes respectively. From a pathological standpoint, note that this condition is not a true neuroma per se. In other words, Morton's neuroma is not a "benign growth of nerve tissue," as any formal definition of neuroma would imply, but rather represents inflammation of the nerve and/or thickening (perineural fibrosis) around it. It is generally agreed that wearing ill-fitted shoes with tapered toe box or high-heels can aggravate this condition.

STRUCTURE AND FUNCTION

The medial and lateral plantar nerves arise from the tibial nerve as it courses from the ankle into the foot, and these go forward to provide sensorimotor innervation to the sole of the foot (Figure 1). The medial plantar nerve is the larger of the two and typically corresponds to innervation of skin and muscle groups along the proximity of the great toe, second, and third toes, as well as the medial side of the fourth. This corresponds to the distribution of the median nerve in the hand. The lateral plantar nerve supplies these components to the lateral half of the fourth toe and the entire plantar aspect of the fifth toe, just as the ulnar nerve does with the fingers. As these nerves course distally, they split into common digital nerves which later, just proximal to each web space near the metatarsal head, bifurcate into the smaller interdigital nerves that branch medially and laterally to enter the respective toes that correspond to the particular interspace from which the nerve came. Unlike the hand, where anastomoses between the median and ulnar nerves are rare, in the foot, the third interdigital nerve is composed of confluent fibers from both the medial and lateral plantar nerves. In about 50-85% of cases, Morton's neuroma affects this third nerve, perhaps owing to its potentially larger size or its location in the foot between the most mobile bony structures. In the remaining cases, the second common digital nerve in the second web space is affected; there is little evidence to suggest any significant degree of involvement to the nerve in the 1st or 4th web space, for reasons that remain unclear.

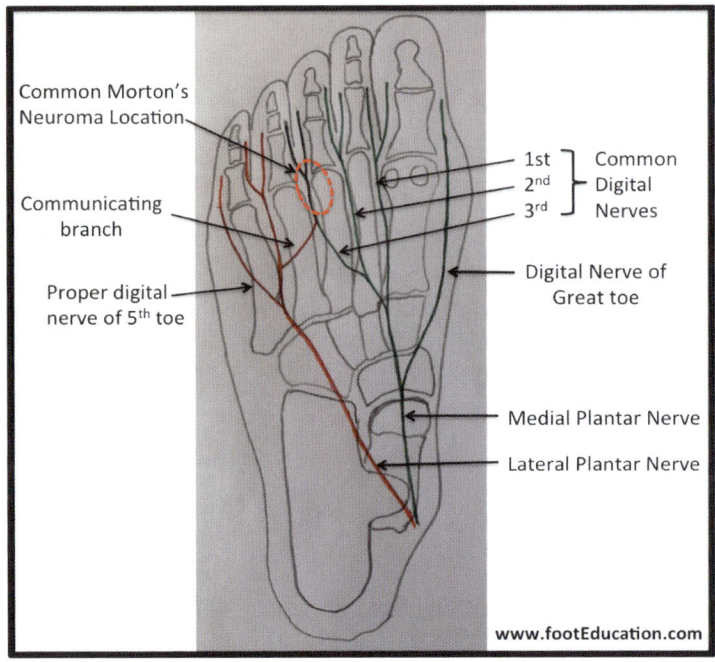

Figure 1: Digital Nerves on the Plantar Aspect of the Foot

Normally, a healthy nerve in one of these interspaces looks like a piece of spaghetti. A true Morton's neuroma is usually inflamed looking and perhaps adherent to the overlying intermetatarsal ligament. The neuroma itself is often directly under the plantar skin, or protected by only a thin layer of subcutaneous tissue (Figure 2). The tissue is usually a pale yellow soft mass. Histologically, there is evidence of fibroblast and Schwann cell proliferation within extensive perivascular and subintimal fibrosis. Additionally, demyelination, axonal damage, and hyalinized nodules (Renaut bodies) are present under the perineurium.

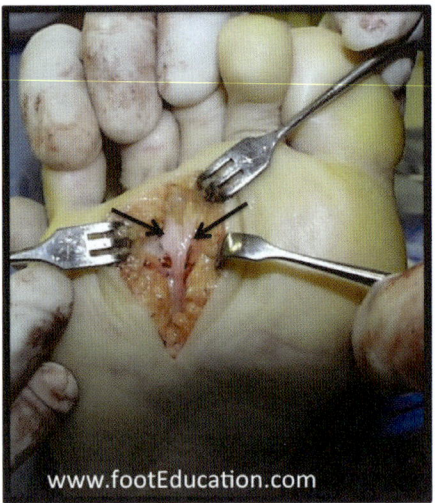

Figure 2. Location of Nerve Directly Under the Skin (between base of 3rd and 4th toes)

The exact etiology of Morton's neuroma is unknown. The eponymous Morton himself suggested that capsulitis of the metatarsophalangeal joint was the source of pain. While the exact etiology of the condition remains unclear, it is believed to be related to localized repetitive overload and irritation of the nerve within the forefoot. Vascular, anatomical, traumatic, systemic, biomechanical, and other proposed pathoetiologies, however, also exist. Betts speculated that the contraction of the flexor digitorum brevis caused the nerve to shear against the intermetatarsal ligament, which in turn caused inflammation. Another theory is that bursal enlargement produces an ischemic effect. Last, some authors have advocated that normal biomechanics alone may be responsible: shearing forces are produced when the relatively mobile 4th metatarsal moves against the relatively fixed 3rd metatarsal, and the nerve may be compressed against the intermetatarsal ligament during the heel-rise phase of gait.

PATIENT PRESENTATION

A patient with a Morton's neuroma often complains of a burning, sharp pain located between the third and fourth toes and worsened with tight fitting shoewear or repetitive loads. The pain is often plantar at the metatarsal heads and radiates distally on either side of the toe; it can also radiate from the forefoot up the leg proximally. In some patients, the pain is alleviated by walking barefoot or taking off shoewear and massaging the foot. Patients may also complain of the sensation of a stone or pebble under the toes or forefoot when walking, and occasionally they will describe an associated intermittent or constant numbness along the involved interspace.

On direct examination, the patient's foot often appears unremarkable, without signs of bursitis, swelling, or other abnormality. On palpation, the usual location of pain is at the interspace between the metatarsal heads. Interdigital skin sensation can be decreased.

A useful test for Morton's neuroma is the "lateral squeeze" or compression test: when the forefoot is compressed by the examiner's hands a painful or palpable "Mulder's click" might be produced by the uncomfortable subluxation of the neuroma between the metatarsal heads.

OBJECTIVE EVIDENCE

There is no one sine qua non test for Morton's neuroma. It is usually a clinical diagnosis, made via consistent findings elucidated thorough history and physical examination. Imaging, however, is necessary to rule out its differential diagnoses. Occasionally, an x-ray may show lateral toe deviation through MTP joint instability or capsulitis, arthritis change in the adjacent joint, or even a stress fracture of a metatarsal. MRI and ultrasound may corroborate Morton's neuroma, but they do not have a terribly high sensitivity or specificity. Injection of local anesthetics may also confirm the diagnosis of a Morton's neuroma by producing rapid (though temporary) amelioration of symptoms.

EPIDEMIOLOGY

The incidence of Morton's neuroma is not known. What is known is the incidence is about 5 times higher in women than in men. The left and right feet are equally affected. The typical patient is about 45 years old.

DIFFERENTIAL DIAGNOSIS

Most chronic pain in the forefoot is NOT the result of a Morton's neuroma. Other more common sources of metatarsalgia (the medical term for forefoot pain) are peripheral neuropathy (from diabetes most likely); stress fractures of the metatarsals; synovitis of the MTP joints, or other inflammation; and trauma. Also, to be considered are Freiberg's infraction (avascular necrosis of the metatarsal head), tarsal tunnel syndrome, infection, and tumors. A thorough physical examination is essential in differentiating among these possible diagnoses.

RED FLAGS

Foot pain in patients with diabetes can be the harbinger of complications. A history of diabetes, thus, should motivate an especially detailed examination.

TREATMENT OPTIONS AND OUTCOMES

Non-operative treatment is the best initial approach. The patient should be instructed to wear shoes with a large toes box and low heels; a metatarsal pad or a custom orthotic can be used to relieve pressure as well. The use of anti-inflammatory medications can be justified empirically, for pain relief. Physical therapy modalities such as ultrasound or electrical stimulation might help but studies demonstrating their effectiveness are lacking. An intermetatarsal injection that perfuses the neurovascular bundle can, with the addition of local anesthetic, help confirm the diagnosis, and a corticosteroid in the cocktail may help produce enduring relief.

If a patient fails to improve with non-operative measures over the passage of time, and if all other potential sources of the pain have been eliminated as diagnostic possibilities, surgery may be indicated. Several treatments are currently employed, including formal resection of the nerve proximal to the area of fibrosis. Another option is simple surgical release of the intermetatarsal ligament and removal of scar tissue. While resection is thought to be more definitive, transecting the nerve results in permanent toe numbness and can result in a troublesome recurrent ('True') neuroma should the remaining stump grow back and become symptomatic. Thus, there remains disagreement as to which operation is best.

Beyond what are considered the standard risks of any orthopaedic procedures, such as infection, wound healing complications, or blood clots, there are a few certain complications that are specific to this procedure and should be noted. These include persistent or worsened pain in the event this is not the cause of the patient's problem or in the case that the nerve stump grows back and becomes bothersome. Complex regional pain syndrome (formerly known as reflex sympathetic dystrophy) can also appear in rare instances. These particular complications are relatively rare, but can be difficult to solve if they occur.

RISK FACTORS AND PREVENTION

There are no clear risk factors since the exact etiology of is unknown. Tight ill-fitting shoes and shoes with high heels likely contribute to the development of Morton's neuroma, and their use should be avoided if possible.

RELATED HISTORICAL INFORMATION

Stigler's Law of Eponymy states that no scientific discovery has ever been named after its original discoverer. Indeed, Stigler's Law was itself described without credit by Robert K. Merton! This law applies here, as this condition is not named for its original discoverer. Although Morton has his name attached to this disorder (by being first to write about the symptoms), it was Betts who first correctly described the pathology. Complicating this eponym, the Dr. Morton whose name bears this pathology was Thomas Morton rather than Dudley Morton, the latter who authored the landmark text, "The Human Foot: It's Evolution, Physiology, and Functional Disorders."

KEY TERMS

Morton's neuroma, Medial and lateral plantar nerves, digital nerves, intermetatarsal ligament, perineural fibrosis, metatarsalgia

SKILLS

Perform a lateral squeeze test and elicit a Mulder's click, described under patient presentation.

CHAPTER 6.

PLANTAR FASCIITIS

DESCRIPTION

Plantar fasciitis is a common source of pain under the heel (Figure 1). The etiology of the condition is thought to be overuse, with traction and shear forces applied to the plantar fascia causing microscopic injuries to the tissue. It is not a purely inflammatory condition as the "itis" suffix would suggest. Classic findings of plantar fasciitis include pain and tenderness in the heel at the junction of the plantar fascia and the medial calcaneal tuberosity. Symptoms are usually worse with the first few steps in the morning (so-called "start up pain"). Helpful treatments include stretching of the calf muscles and the plantar fascia itself and the use of orthotics with a medial arch support.

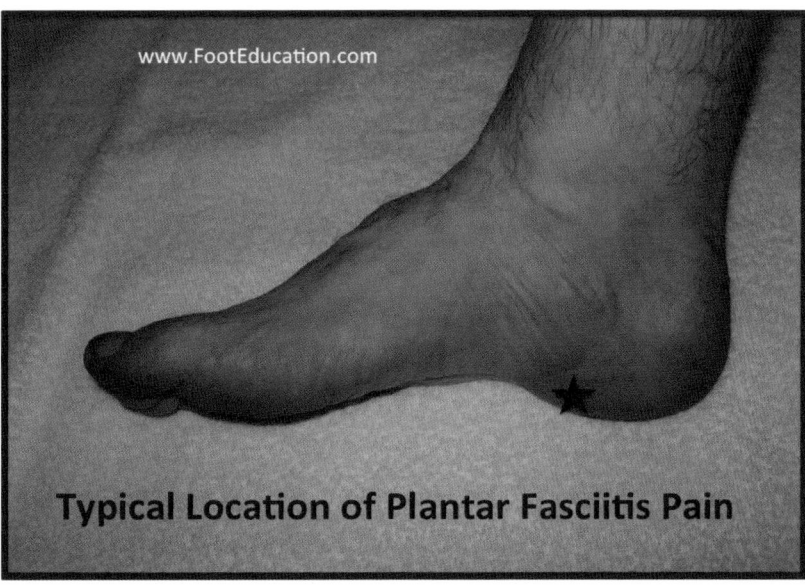

Figure 1: Common Location of Pain in Plantar Fasciitis

STRUCTURE AND FUNCTION

The plantar fascia is a sheet of fibrous tissue (technically termed an aponeurosis) running along the sole of the foot from the calcaneus to the base of the proximal phalanges, with fibers merging with the dermis, transverse metatarsal ligaments, and flexor tendon sheaths as well. The plantar fascia is mostly inelastic, with minimal elongation.

Weight-bearing forces tend to flatten the medial longitudinal arch as forces are applied to the foot. The plantar fascia prevents this collapse, by maintaining the distance between the calcaneus and the metatarsals. Note that the insertion of the plantar fascia is on the toes; hence dorsiflexion of the toes pulls on the plantar fascia, winding it under the metatarsals and thereby elevating the arch, a so-called "windlass" effect.

Plantar fasciitis is thought to be produced by overuse, creating a chronic microscopic injury to the plantar-medial origin of the plantar fascia. A heel spur is commonly found on x-ray, but is neither a sensitive nor specific finding. Only 50% of patients with heel pain will have heel spurs and about 15% of people with asymptomatic feet will have them. Accordingly, it is likely that the spur is not causing the condition. Further, cadaveric dissections have demonstrated that the spur from the calcaneus is within the flexor tendons, rather than the plantar fascia itself.

Histologic findings in plantar fasciitis includes tears in the fascia, myxoid degeneration, angiofibroblastic hyperplasia, and collagen necrosis and not inflammation per se. However, inflammation could be part of the healing process.

PATIENT PRESENTATION

Healing of micro-trauma is thought to cause tightening of the plantar fascia when the patient is at rest, especially as the foot and ankle assume a plantarflexed position at night. Upon ambulation, when the foot and ankle forced into a neutral and dorsiflexed position, the healing tissue is strained. Thus, the classic presentation of plantar fasciitis as an especially sharp pain with the first few steps in the morning or after prolonged rest. This pain is localized to the plantar medial aspect of the calcaneal tuberosity (Figure 1). It will often improve after some movement or stretching. However, it will tend to recur and worsen as the day progresses, particularly if the patient has had prolonged periods of significant weight-bearing activities such as walking or standing.

The foot and ankle physical exam should include inspection of the patient's stance, foot shape, and gait; full neurologic evaluation; and identification of any areas of tenderness, especially at the medial plantar aspect of the heel. In some patients, dorsiflexion of the toes may exacerbate the pain via the windlass effect.

OBJECTIVE EVIDENCE

Plantar fasciitis is diagnosed by history and physical examination, but x-rays may help rule out other diagnoses. A lateral weight-bearing view of the foot will often demonstrate a calcaneal heel spur, though this should be considered an incidental finding. As previously noted the presence of a heel spur does not directly correlate with symptoms.

Diagnosis of classic plantar fasciitis requires only a good history and physical exam. However, in atypical presentations or when symptoms are recalcitrant and other diagnoses are being considered, further imaging studies may be indicated. An MRI or a triple-phase bone scan can differentiate plantar fasciitis from a calcaneal stress fracture – a much less common cause of heel pain. An MRI may also be used to rule out other uncommon causes of heel pain such as tumors and infection. Ultrasound is less expensive than an MRI and provides no radiation exposure but requires specific expertise that many physicians lack. Typical ultrasound findings include a thickened, hypoechoic plantar fascia with soft-tissue edema.

Except in rare instances where an inflammatory condition is suspected, laboratory studies are not indicated in the workup of patients with plantar heel pain. Similarly, in the uncommon situation where neurological symptoms are suspected, nerve conduction studies may help exclude local nerve entrapment (medial plantar nerve).

EPIDEMIOLOGY

Plantar fasciitis is the most common cause of heel pain. Patients are usually 40-50 years of age. Plantar fasciitis may be bilateral in some patients although one heel is usually more painful than the other.

DIFFERENTIAL DIAGNOSIS

Plantar fasciitis is the most likely cause of heel pain but other entities such as overload heel pain syndrome, heel pad atrophy, entrapment of the first branch of the lateral plantar nerve (Baxter's nerve), tarsal tunnel syndrome, calcaneal stress fracture and seronegative inflammatory disease can also lead to heel pain.

Patients with overload heel pain syndrome will have pain that is centrally located in the heel rather than towards the inside of the heel pad such as is typical in plantar fasciitis. Certain foot patterns such as high arched feet, relative weakness of the calf muscle, or dysfunction of the Achilles tendon may be predisposed to overloading the heel with resulting symptoms.

Marked pain after a sudden increase in the patient's level of activity or training should prompt a work-up to rule out a calcaneal stress fracture. Infection or neoplasm are more likely when the plantar heel pain is present at night, especially when accompanied by unplanned weight loss, fevers or chills. These are, in general, unlikely diagnoses.

Burning pain is not typical of plantar fasciitis and may suggest nerve irritation as a source of the pain: Baxter's neuritis (compression of the first branch of the lateral plantar nerve, also known as the inferior calcaneal nerve); peripheral neuropathy or radiculopathy.

RED FLAGS

Any deviation from the classic history for plantar fasciitis should be a red flag to consider other diagnoses.

TREATMENT OPTIONS AND OUTCOMES

The vast majority of patients will have their symptoms resolve with or without treatment over a period of 6 months. Recovery can be accelerated with a program of calf and plantar fascia stretching, activity modification to avoid precipitating activities, and comfort shoewear. Formal physical therapy, immobilization via cast or boot, steroid injections, and rarely extracorporeal shock wave therapy may also be employed.

A plantar fascia specific stretching program is highly beneficial in treating plantar fasciitis (Figure 2). This is performed by gently pulling the ankle and toes into dorsiflexion. This produces tension in the plantar fascia. The stretch position should be held for 10 seconds and repeated 10 times. The timing of when this is performed is important. It should be done prior to the first step in the morning and during the day before standing after prolonged inactivity.

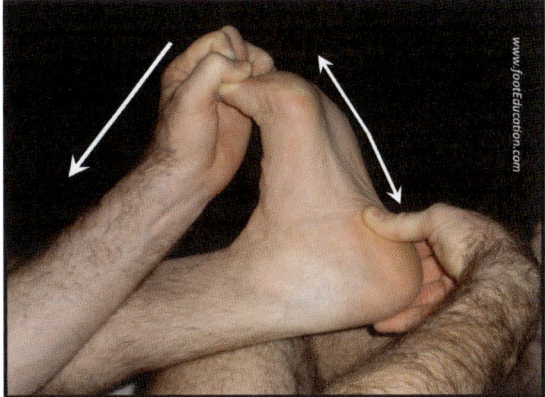

Figure 2: Plantar Fascia Specific Stretch

Calf stretching should be performed with the knee straight so that the gastrocnemius (which originates on the femur) is stretched. It is also important to internally rotate the foot to lock out the subtalar joint during the stretch. For patients with plantar fasciitis it is usually best to ask them to rotate their foot inward with the heel on the ground until the heel pain diminishes, then stretch. Six sets of 30 seconds per side done daily is recommended.

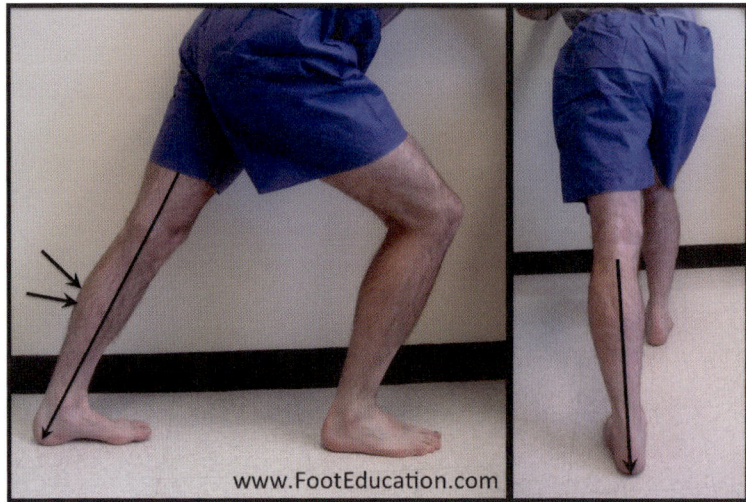

Figure 3. Calf (Gastrocnemius) Stretch (left leg). Note that the back knee is straight and the back foot is internally rotated.

With resolution of the heel pain symptoms, it is important to continue calf stretching and plantar fascia stretching on a semi-regular basis so as to minimize the risk of recurrence.

Any activity that has recently been started, such as a new running routine or a new exercise at the gym that may have increased loading through the heel area, should be stopped on a temporary basis until the symptoms have resolved. At that point, these activities can be gradually started again.

A soft, over-the-counter orthotic with an accommodating arch support might be helpful. Evidence supporting the need for a custom orthotic is lacking. Shoes with a stiff sole and rocker-bottom contour off-load the plantar fascia at its origin and likewise may be effective.

Anti-inflammatory medication may ameliorate symptoms. Corticosteroid Injection can give temporary relief but may lead to atrophy of the fat pad. Injections of preparations of autologous blood (ex. plasma rich protein – PRP) have been described but lack high quality supportive evidence.

A plantar fascia night splint (Figure 4) that keeps the ankle in a neutral position, perpendicular to the foot, while the patient sleeps, can be helpful in alleviating the significant morning symptoms. Avoiding the position of plantar flexion can prevent some of the shortening of the fascia that occurs at night.

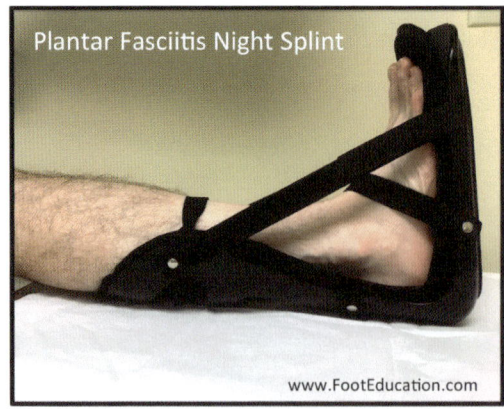

Figure 4. Plantar Fasciitis Night Splint

Surgery is rarely indicated in the treatment of plantar fasciitis. Only patients who have persistent symptoms despite adhering to the non-operative treatment for a minimum of 6 months should be considered for surgery. Endoscopic or open partial plantar fasciotomy involves removal of the injured area of the plantar fascia. Although this procedure has produced good results in some cases, complete release of the plantar fascia may lead to a flat foot and chronic foot pain. Therefore, it is recommended that less than 40% of the plantar fascia be released (though an appropriately conservative release may limit the effectiveness of the procedures).

A surgical recession of the gastrocnemius (ex. Strayer procedure) theoretically should help resolve the symptoms associated with plantar fasciitis, as gastrocnemius contracture is a known risk factor for the development plantar fasciitis. There are only limited studies assessing the long-term effectiveness of this procedure.

RISK FACTORS AND PREVENTION

Risk factors for plantar fasciitis include a job or lifestyle associated with prolonged standing, excessive body weight, increasing age, a change in activity level, Achilles tightness, and a stiff calf muscle (gastrocnemius). A flat foot or a high arch deformity (pes planus and pes cavus, respectively) can increase loading of the plantar fascia and increase the risk of developing plantar fasciitis. However, any foot type can develop this condition.

MISCELLANY

Fascia and political Fascism are related words. A fascia is of course connective tissue, typically that wraps around muscle fibers. Fascism comes from the Italian word *fasci*, political groups or guild, itself derived from the Latin word *fascis*, meaning "bundle."

KEY TERMS

plantar fascia, plantar fasciitis, calcaneus, Achilles tendon

SKILLS

Learn how to instruct patients on stretching the plantar fascia and gastrocnemius.

CHAPTER 7.

TENDON DISORDERS OF THE FOOT AND ANKLE

DESCRIPTION

Important tendons cross the anterior, medial and lateral aspects of the ankle. These include, respectively, the tibialis anterior; the tibialis posterior; and the pair of peroneal tendons (peroneus longus and brevis). Due to their important roles during gait, each of these tendons may be subject to overuse and inflammation. When symptoms of inflammation are present, the clinical diagnosis of tendonitis may apply. The large Achilles tendon runs posterior to the ankle and inserts into the calcaneus. It may be affected by a number of clinical conditions that are reviewed in chapter 8 (Achilles tendon disorders) and chapter 14 (Achilles tendon rupture).

The terminology of tendon disorders may be confusing. (Indeed, the first hit on Google for the term "tendonitis" takes you to a site about "tendinitis.") Although it is certainly acceptable to use "Tendinopathy" as an all-encompassing term denoting a disease of a tendon, it may be helpful to think of three distinct disorders:

Tendonitis, also known as Tendinitis, refers to a painful clinical condition where there is acute pain and swelling due to microtearing of the tendon and the resulting inflammatory response.

Tendonosis (or tendinosis) is a chronic degenerative condition in which repetitive overuse and aging leads to a non-inflammatory degeneration of the tendon's collagen over time.

Paratenonitis is an inflammation of the lining of the thin lining of connective tissue that surrounds many tendons allowing the tendon to glide more easily, namely the paratenon.

In a nutshell, you must ask: is the problem an acute inflammatory problem, or is this a degenerative condition? Or is the problem extrinsic to the tendon altogether?

Note that it can be difficult at times to differentiate clinically between these three conditions. Many cases of acute inflammatory tendonitis occur in the setting of underlying degenerative changes within the tissue. Therefore, while the term tendonitis will be used broadly in this chapter, it should be kept in mind that the described condition may not be tendonitis, per se.

STRUCTURE AND FUNCTION

The tibialis anterior muscle is the most medial muscle of the anterior compartment of the leg (Figure 1). It stabilizes the ankle as the foot hits the ground during the contact phase of walking and dorsiflexes the ankle to help the foot clear the ground during the swing phase. It also provides half of the force needed to 'lock' the ankle, as would be needed to kick a ball, for example: by providing an isometric contraction against its antagonists, the soleus and gastrocnemius, the tibio-talar joint is held in a fixed position.

The tibialis posterior muscle belly originates on the posterior aspects of the tibia and fibula and the tendon crosses behind the medial malleolus to insert primarily on the navicular (Figure 2). It actively inverts the foot and also plantar flexes the ankle, but its primary role is to support the medial arch of the foot. Contraction of the tibialis posterior locks the joints of the midfoot during gait progression to create a rigid lever in the foot. Therefore, rupture or even stretching of this tendon can lead to flat feet.

The peroneus longus and brevis muscle bellies originate on the fibula and the tendons course together along the bone, with the brevis medial to the longus (Figure 3). They cross the ankle behind the lateral malleolus, in a groove covered by the superior peroneal retinaculum. The peroneus longus tendon then continues in a plantar direction along the sole of the foot to the base of the first metatarsal bone. The peroneus brevis tendon inserts into a tuberosity at the base of the fifth metatarsal bone, on its lateral side. The peroneus muscles plantarflex and everts the foot.

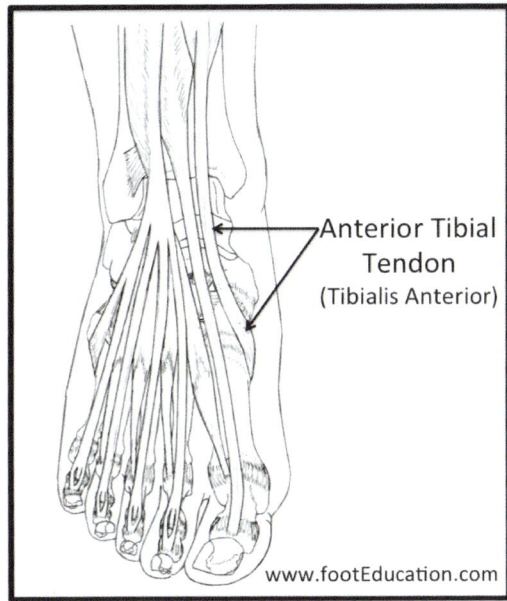

Figure 1: Tibialis Anterior Tendon

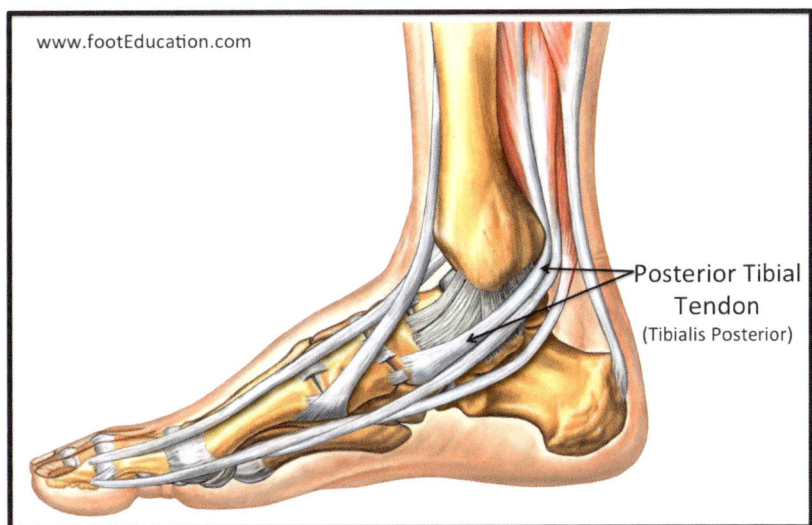

Figure 2: Tibialis Posterior Tendon

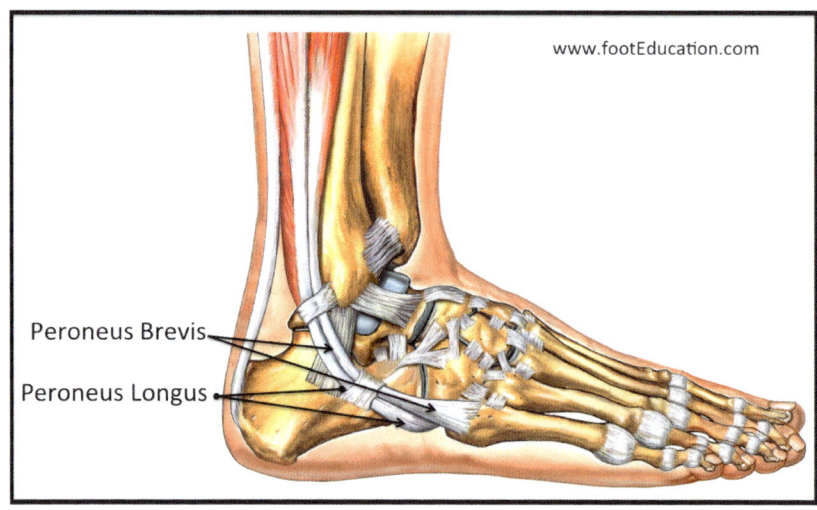

Figure 3: Tendons of the Peroneus Longus and Brevis

PATIENT PRESENTATION

Tibialis Anterior tendonitis leads to pain and often swelling in the front of the ankle and into the medial midfoot (Figure 4). Symptoms typically occur in middle aged and older individuals. They often occur after prolonged exercise or ankle injury, and can be related to change in activity levels or footwear. Symptoms are aggravated by standing and walking and alleviated by rest. Examination will often reveal tenderness and sometimes swelling over the anterior aspect of the ankle. Resisted dorsiflexion of the ankle against the examiner's hand will often exacerbate symptoms.

Tibialis Posterior tendonitis presents as medial ankle and arch pain, worsened with prolonged standing and often in conjunction with a flat foot and prominent navicular bone on the medial aspect of the foot. Pain with resisted inversion and tenderness along the course of the tendon to its insertion on the navicular are hallmarks of this condition. If there is tenderness at the insertion but not along the course of the tendon, a symptomatic *accessory navicular* may be present. This can be confirmed with a radiograph.

The integrity of the Tibialis Posterior can be assessed with a *single leg heel rise*; having the patient stand up on the ball of the foot, with the contralateral foot off the ground entirely (that is, in a stork position). When viewed from behind, the intact tendon will be seen to invert the ankle and heel. A lack of this motion suggests tendon dysfunction or failure. Note: that if the contralateral foot is kept on the ground and helps the patient stand on his or her toes, that assistance might prevent the tested tibialis posterior from generating enough force to invert the ankle, and the test can be falsely negative. Note also that some patients with severe tendonopathy may simply be unable to stand on one leg at all. This can be related to pain, weakness, or a combination of the two.

Patients with *peroneal tendonitis* present with pain and, occasionally, swelling near the posterolateral ankle (Figure 5). Resisted eversion will produce pain. Concomitant sural nerve irritation (by inflamed or damaged tendon) can lead to either decreased sensation or a burning over the lateral or outside aspect of the foot. There may be pain at the insertion of the brevis on the metatarsal, and if there was an acute event precipitating the pain, an x-ray should be obtained to exclude a bone injury.

With an injury to the retinaculum, the peroneal tendons may be free to slip in and out of their normal position behind the fibula bone at the level of the ankle joint. This condition is known as *chronic subluxating peroneal tendonitis*. Patients with this condition might describe a snapping sensation with activity; the subluxation can at times be reproduced on physical exam.

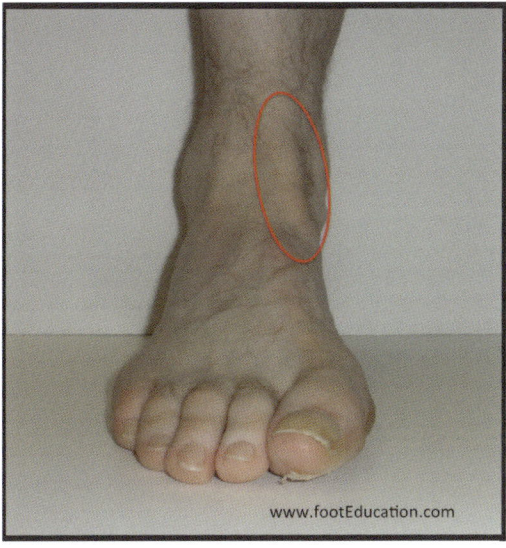

Figure 4: Location of pain and swelling in tibialis anterior tendonitis

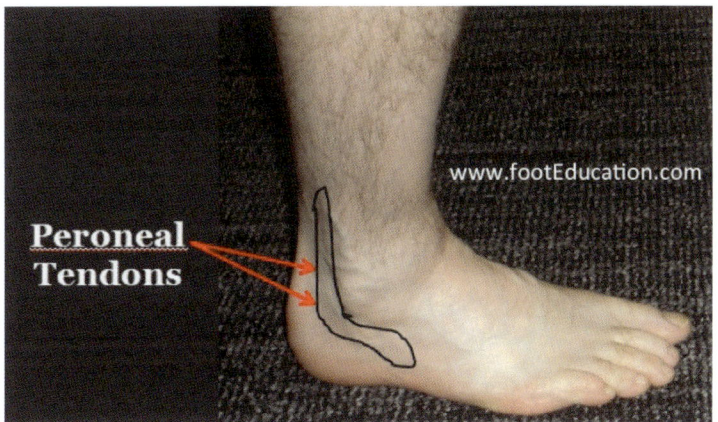

Figure 5: Location of pain and swelling in peroneal tendonitis

OBJECTIVE EVIDENCE

Suspected tibialis anterior tendonitis can be evaluated with plain x-rays of the foot and ankle which might reveal bone injury or arthrosis in the ankle or midfoot joints.

Posterior tibial tendon disorders may be studied with weight-bearing x-rays of the foot to assess the extent of the flatfoot deformity, if any. Plain x-rays may also reveal an accessory navicular or a tarsal coalition. MRI can show damage to the tendon, injury to ankle ligaments, and identify arthrosis in the joints of the hindfoot.

In the case of suspected peroneal tendonitis, plain weight-bearing x-rays are likely to show evidence of a high arched foot pattern, but the main goal of radiographs is to exclude a fracture of the fifth metatarsal, bony prominences that can irritate the tendons or lateral ankle arthrosis. An MRI can determine if there is tearing or tenosynovitis of the peroneal tendons.

EPIDEMIOLOGY

Although the incidence of ankle tendonitis has not been measured, anecdotal evidence suggests that posterior tibial and peroneal tendonitis are relatively common. Whereas anterior tibial tendonitis is less common, except perhaps in younger athletes who have just increased training regiments or started running up and down hills (PMID: 19912714). Risk factors for peroneal tendon problems include a high arch foot with an inward (varus) heel and can occur at any age. Tibialis posterior problems are associated with a flatfoot deformity and more commonly occur in patients in their 40s and 50s

DIFFERENTIAL DIAGNOSIS

Anterior ankle pain, similar to that of tendonitis, is more commonly caused by ankle arthritis or anterior ankle impingement.

Lateral ankle pain may be caused by ankle sprains, sural nerve irritation, fracture of the anterior process of the calcaneus, or fracture of the base of the fifth metatarsal (e.g., Jones fracture). Radiographs can also demonstrate a calcification within the peroneus longus tendon called "painful os peroneum syndrome" or POPS.

Medial ankle pain near the posterior tibialis can be due to an accessory navicular, spring ligament injury, or medial malleolar stress fracture. Posterior tibial dysfunction can be seen in rheumatoid arthritis.

RED FLAGS

Pain along the course of the tibialis posterior may suggest attritional tearing of the tendon. This should be detected and treated before the tendon ruptures, which could cause an acquired flatfoot. Persistent tenderness on the lateral aspect of the ankle can be related to fractures of the anterior process of the calcaneus, base of fifth metatarsal, or cuboid. Radiographs can help rule these out.

TREATMENT OPTIONS AND OUTCOMES

Patients with ankle tendonitis can often be treated successfully non-operatively. Modalities include topical and oral anti-inflammatory medication, icing, ankle bracing, activity modification, physical therapy, an orthotic, and avoidance of precipitating activity with sudden cutting or changes of direction.

In patients with posterior tendon dysfunction and an associated flatfoot deformity (*acquired adult flatfoot deformity*), it may be necessary to perform some type of a flatfoot reconstruction if non-operative treatment fails. This usually includes a transfer of another tendon (usually the flexor digitorum longus) to support the arch combined with a bony procedure, such as a medializing calcaneal osteotomy, to address the associated foot deformity. Removing an accessory navicular and reattaching the tendon (Kidner procedure) may be necessary in patients with a painful recalcitrant accessory navicular.

In patients with a large peroneal tendon tear or a bony prominence that abrades the tendon, surgical repair with resection of the irritant may be beneficial. A small peroneal tendon tear that does not respond to non-operative treatment may also benefit from debrided and repaired.

RISK FACTORS AND PREVENTION

Risk factors for *peroneal tendonitis* include overuse and a high arched foot. An orthotic with a lateral heel post and a recessed area under the first metatarsal head may be useful if a patient has a cavus (high arched) foot pattern.

Risk factors for *tibialis anterior tendonitis* include tight calves, obesity, flatfeet, and overuse.

Rheumatoid conditions predispose to joint capsular laxity and tendon attenuation and may cause posterior tendon dysfunction.

MISCELLANY

Patients with Charcot-Marie-Tooth disease, an inherited neuromuscular disorder, have asymmetrical residual weakness of the foot and ankle muscles, with the peroneus longus attaching to the base of the first metatarsal, relatively spared. The unopposed pull of this muscle against its weakened natural antagonist (tibialis anterior) causes the classic deformity of marked cavus (high arches), as shown in Figure 6.

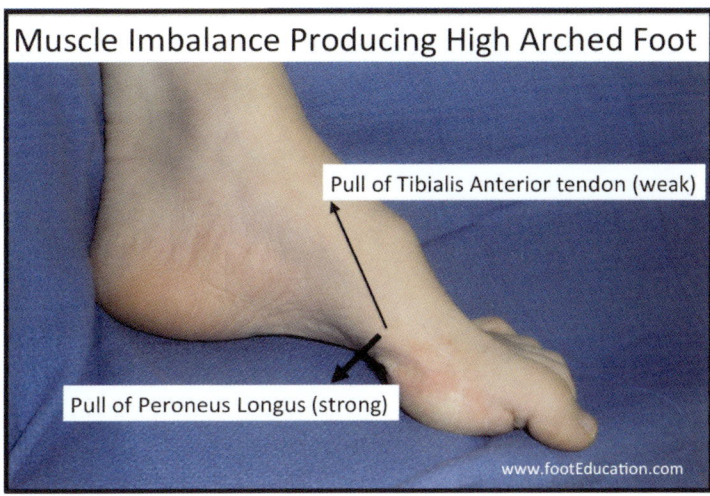

Figure 6: The unopposed pull of the peroneus longus causes the classic deformity of Charcot-Marie-Tooth disease, namely, marked cavus of the foot.

KEY TERMS

Tendonitis; tendinitis, tendonosis, tendinosis, tendinpathy, inflammation; tibialis anterior; peroneus longus; peroneus brevis; posterior tibial tendonitis, acquired adult flatfoot deformity; accessory navicular

SKILLS

Identify the surface anatomy of the tendons themselves, as well as the navicular, 5th metatarsal, and lateral retinaculum. Perform resistance tests for each tendon to determine strength, function, and pain that may be related to tendon injury or other pathology. Perform and interpret the single leg heel rise test. Recognize an incipient posterior tendon rupture. Identify fractures and other disorders on radiographic images

CHAPTER 8.

ACHILLES TENDON DISORDERS

DESCRIPTION

The Achilles tendon is subject to high forces with each step and therefore subject to wear-and-tear damage. There are many pathological conditions that affect the Achilles tendon, but the most common chronic conditions are tendonitis and bursitis. The most common acute condition is an Achilles rupture (often superimposed on wear-and-tear).

STRUCTURE AND FUNCTION

The Achilles tendon is the largest and strongest tendon in the human body. It attaches the posterior calf muscles (the gastrocnemius and soleus) to the calcaneus.

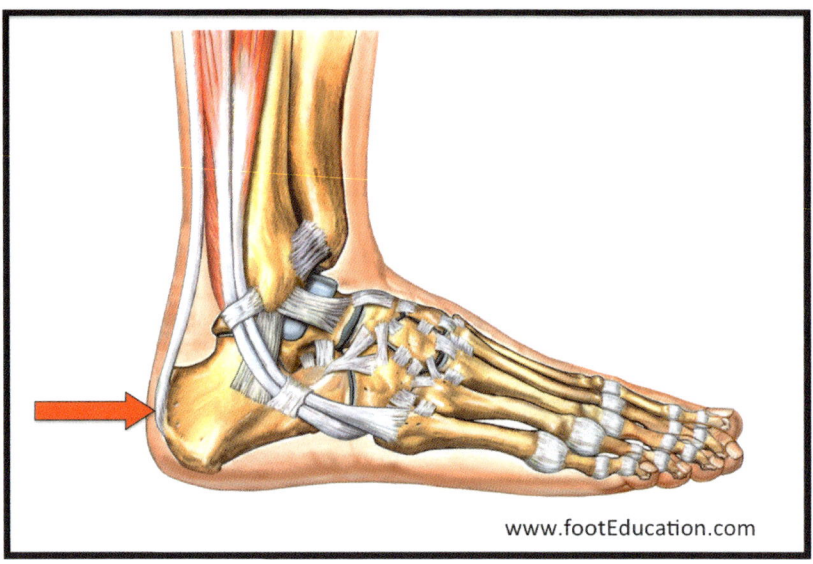

Figure 1: The Insertion of the Achilles Tendon (red arrow)

The posterior calf muscles both actively plantar flex the ankle and resist passive dorsiflexion during walking, jumping, and running. Note that when the person places the ball of his or her foot on the ground during gait, body weight and momentum will force the ankle into dorsiflexion. Resisting this motion, and in turn decelerating the landing of the heel, is powered by the posterior calf muscles. Forces up to 3 times body weight may be applied to the tendon when this happens while walking; even greater forces are applied while jumping and running. The Achilles tendon inserts into the posterior surface of the calcaneus. The insertion begins about halfway between the plantar and superior surface of the calcaneus (Figure 1).

A bursa lies between the tendon and calcaneus above the insertion point: the so-called retrocalcaneal bursa. Another bursa lies posterior to the tendon between the tendon and skin, namely, the subcutaneous calcaneal bursa. A bursa is a fluid-filled sac (the word shares its origin with the English word "purse") that normally exists between tendons and bone in places where the bone surface may be prominent; this allows the tendon to glide more easily. In the healthy state, the bursa is only a few cells thick, and the bursa is filled with only a small amount of lubricating fluid. However, when irritated, a bursa can become markedly thickened and filled with larger amounts of fluid. This condition is known as bursitis.

PATIENT PRESENTATION

Achilles tendonitis is a chronic condition characterized by pain and swelling in the Achilles tendon.

Symptoms of tendonitis are produced by swelling and inflammation of the tissue that surrounds the Achilles tendon – the paratendon. As such, the condition may be more appropriately described as an Achilles tenosynovitis (inflammation of the lining surrounding the Achilles tendon). Inflammation of the tendon can be caused either by direct pressure from shoewear or more commonly, as part of the healing response to over-use and micro-trauma.

There are two types of Achilles tendonitis: non-insertional tendonitis and insertional tendonitis.

Achilles Tendonitis (Non-Insertional):

In classic non-insertional (or mid-substance) Achilles tendonitis, the pathology is typically located 2 to 6 cm proximal to the insertion of the Achilles tendon to the calcaneus.

Non-insertional Achilles tendonitis is often associated with a history of increased activity level (e.g., starting a new training regimen or attempting to resume a normal activity level after an injury and enforced immobilization).

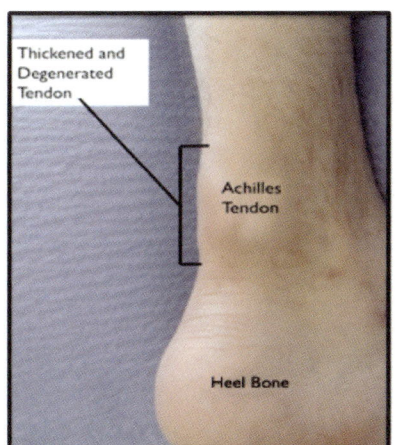 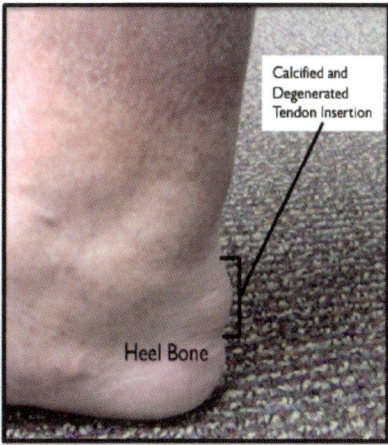

Figure 2: Location of Symptoms: Non-insertional Achilles (Left) and Insertional Achilles (right)

A patient presenting with non-insertional Achilles tendonitis (Figure 2 left) will often describe pain and tenderness 2-6 cm from the insertion of the tendon into the calcaneus. The patient will often describe an increase in activity, such as starting a new training regimen or attempting to resume a normal activity level after an injury to another part of the foot or ankle.

Physical Examination will usually reveal swelling and tenderness around the Achilles tendon. There is often an associated tight calf muscle (equinus contracture). The location of the pain can help differentiate this from insertional tendinitis (Figure 2 right) which presents with pain more distally.

Insertional Achilles Tendonitis:

In so-called "insertional" Achilles tendonitis, the pathology is located at the insertion of the Achilles tendon to the calcaneus (Figure 2, right). Insertional Achilles tendonitis is a product of wear and tear at the attachment ("insertion") of the tendon onto the calcaneus. This degeneration incites an inflammatory response and produces pain at the back of the heel. Eventually, the inflamed Achilles tendon may become calcified, forming bone-like fragments in the tendon.

The pathology associated with insertional Achilles tendonitis includes the "terrible triad" (Figure 3):

1. Degeneration of the Achilles tendon near the insertion site,
2. An inflamed retrocalcaneal bursitis, and
3. A Haglund's deformity (a prominent bony lump on the heel)

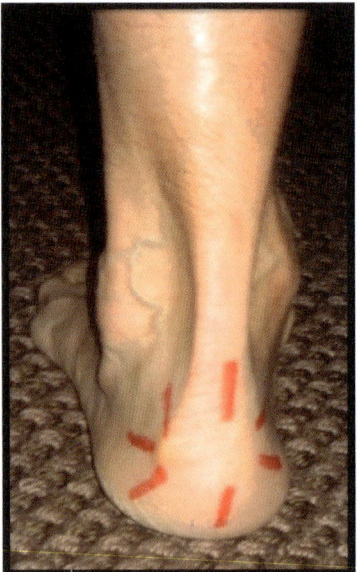

Figure 3: Location of pain in patients with the "Terrible Triad": insertional Achilles tendonitis, retrocalcaneal bursitis, and a prominent bony lump on the heel (known as a Haglund's deformity).

A Haglund's deformity is a bony prominence associated with the upper part of the calcaneus (Figure 4). This is sometimes called a "pump bump." This prominent bone tends to form gradually over many years, and can eventually cause irritation by disrupting nearby structures, including the retrocalcaneal bursa and the Achilles tendon. The bony prominence also creates discomfort by rubbing up against the back of footwear, the so-called "heel counter" of the shoe.

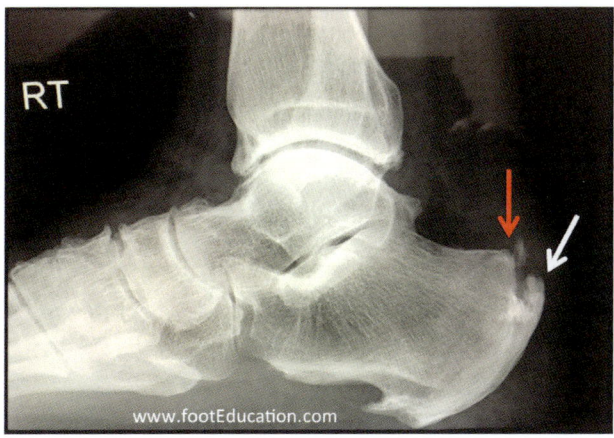

Figure 4: Haglund's Deformity. An x-ray showing both a Haglund's deformity (red arrow) as well as calcification of the Achilles tendon insertion (white arrow)

When a Haglund's deformity is present, the retrocalcaneal bursa can become inflamed. This inflammation can result in exquisite tenderness along the posterior aspect of the heel.

OBJECTIVE EVIDENCE

X-rays will usually be negative in cases of non-insertional Achilles tendonitis, unless there is calcification of the Achilles tendon. (Calcification is relatively rare except in older patients.) Cases of insertional Achilles tendonitis may reveal a calcaneal spur on x-ray.

An MRI can give a detailed view of the soft tissue (Figure 5). However, this test is not routinely indicated in the initial assessment of Achilles tendonitis.

Ultrasound is usually less expensive than an MRI, but may not be available in all settings. Further, use of ultrasound may be limited by the examiner's lack of skill or experience.

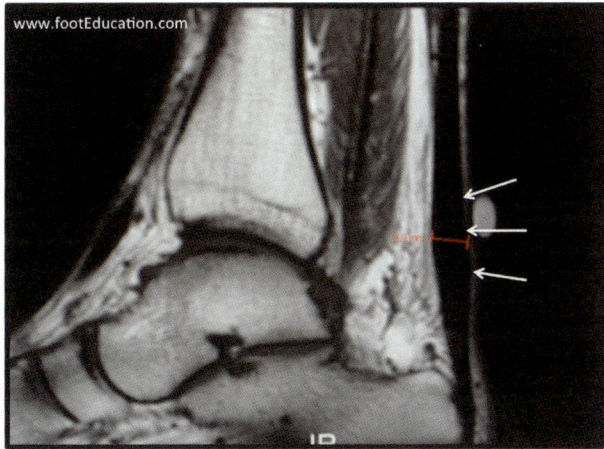

Figure 5: MRI of Achilles Tendonitis (non-insertional) Swelling associated with non-insertional Achilles tendonitis as seen on MRI. The tendon is shown in continuity but is abnormally thickened.

EPIDEMIOLOGY

Insertional Achilles tendonitis with its associated "terrible triad" of heel pain typically occurs in middle-aged individuals who are overweight, though a variant of this condition is also seen in young, active runners. The exact incidence of this bimodal distribution has not been recorded.

Non-Insertional Achilles tendonitis is often associated with an increase in activity level/overuse and tends to occur in patients in their 30s and 40s. According to Jarvinen et al., the reported annual incidence of Achilles tendonitis is between 7-9% in top-level runners (PMID: 15922917).

DIFFERENTIAL DIAGNOSIS

There are four common causes for pain near the back of the heel:

1. non-insertional Achilles tendonitis,
2. insertional Achilles tendonitis (with or without bursitis)
3. paratendonitis (inflammation of the sheath surrounding the Achilles tendon, rather than of the tendon itself), and
4. Achilles tendon rupture.

The Thompson test will identify an Achilles tendon rupture. The precise location of the pain should distinguish non-insertional Achilles tendonitis vs insertional Achilles tendonitis.

RED FLAGS

Although corticosteroid injections in and around the Achilles can be helpful in the short-term managing symptoms they weaken the tendon and predispose to tearing. Be alert for patients that have had corticosteroid injections in this area.

Patients with inflammatory arthropathies may also get inflammation in the lining around their Achilles. If a patient has other joints that are painful or swollen, especially if they are of recent onset, an inflammatory etiology should be ruled out.

TREATMENT OPTIONS AND OUTCOMES

Non-operative Treatment of Achilles Tendonitis

Most patients with Achilles tendonitis can have their symptoms treated effectively without surgery. Insertional Achilles tendonitis can be more recalcitrant to treatment than non-insertional Achilles tendonitis. An initial period of relative rest to allow the symptoms to settle is often beneficial. This is followed by a gradual return to normal activities incorporating the following non-operative treatment elements:

1. Activity modification,
2. Shoewear modification (a heel lift will unload the tendon),
3. Weight Loss (if applicable)
4. Anti-inflammatory medication (if not contra-indicated) and;
5. A rehabilitation program including specific stretching and strengthening exercises.

Stretching the gastrocnemius (outer calf muscle) with the knee straight (Figure 6) is an important component of non-operative treatment. A tight calf muscle will increase the force going through the Achilles tendon and predispose the tendon to micro-tearing.

A graduated eccentric loading program (strengthening the calf muscle while it is lengthening) is an important component of non-operative treatment for non-insertional Achilles tendonitis (Figure 7). However, it may be too aggressive for patients with insertional Achilles tendonitis.

Using a heel lift reduces the "stretch" on the Achilles during walking and thereby reduces the stress on the tendon.

The forces applied to the Achilles tendon during activities are proportional to body weight. Therefore losing weight (even a small amount) can be very helpful.

Surgical Treatment of Achilles Tendonitis

Surgical debridement, that is, the removal of the damaged tissue with meticulous repair of the remaining tendon, may be chosen if non-operative treatment fails. One setting where surgery may be considered more readily is that of a high-level athlete with insertional Achilles tendonitis and a Haglund's deformity. This surgery usually involves removing the prominent excess bone and the thickened inflamed retrocalcaneal bursa and debriding the Achilles tendon. In older, heavy-set middle-aged patients with insertional Achilles tendonitis that have truly failed a focused non-operative treatment regiment it may be necessary to transfer the Flexor Hallucis Longus (FHL) tendon into the calcaneus to help offload the Achilles.

Recovery from surgery can be prolonged. Initially, the leg is immobilized to allow the wound to heal. Once the wound is healed, gentle range of motion exercises can be started. Some patients are limited in weight-bearing for the first six weeks during the healing process. Gradually, activity can be increased. Improvement in strength continues for several months and may take over one year.

Stiffness of the ankle, rupture of the tendon, and deep vein thrombosis are known potential complications of surgery. Wound healing issues and infection can occur and when they do it is a very serious problem because loss of skin and soft-tissue in this area is very hard to treat.

RISK FACTORS AND PREVENTION

Regular calf stretching (Figures 6 & 7), can help improve the Achilles tendon's mechanical compliance ("stretchability" in layman's terms) and makes it more resilient.

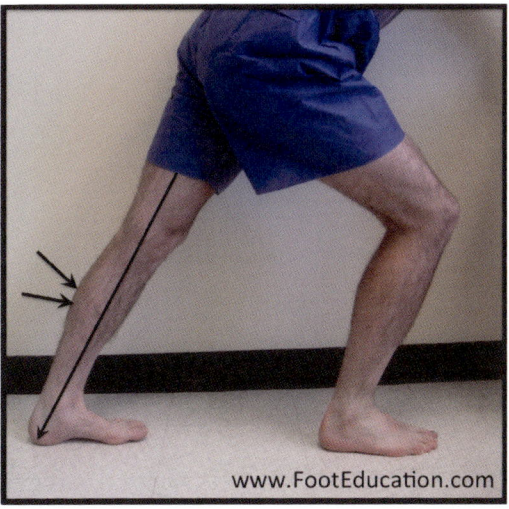

Figure 6: Calf Stretching

A consistent calf-stretching program is an important part of treatment and prevention of Achilles injuries (Figure 6). Leaning against the wall with one foot forward and the back heel kept on the ground will stretch the Achilles and posterior calf muscles. As it is the outer calf muscle (gastrocnemius) that is usually tight this stretch should be performed with the knee straight as the gastrocnemius originates from the posterior aspect of the distal femur. Bending the knee will take the tension off the gastrocnemius and place it on the soleus.

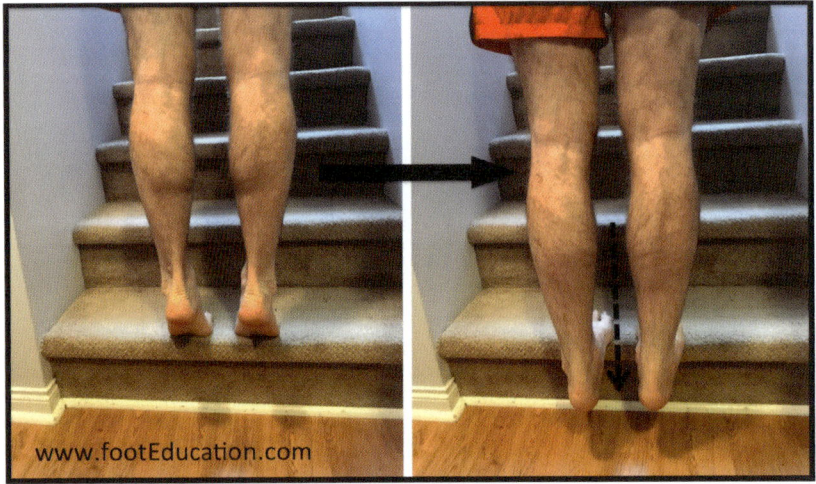

Figure 7: Eccentric Calf Stretching and Strengthening

Controlled "eccentric" exercises where the Achilles tendon is being lengthened while the calf muscle contracts, may help prevent (or treat) Achilles tendonitis (Figure 7). This includes exercises such as the "Heel drop" shown here. In this exercise, patients stand on their toes while positioned on the edge of a ledge such as a stair. They then slowly lower their heels down below the ledge simultaneously stretching and strengthening the Achilles tendon. This can be done with both legs at a time (bilaterally) or for a more concentrated effort, one leg at a time. It can also be done with the knees straight (putting force on the gastrocnemius) or the knees bent (putting force on the soleus). Patients should gradually work up to performing 5 sets of 10 repetitions. These exercises should be performed 5-6 days per week during the active treatment phase and then 3 times per week to minimize the chance of developing recurrent symptoms. It is critical that this exercise is approached cautiously, as it has the potential to put excessive pressure on the Achilles. Patients should always warm up first (ex. get their blood flowing on an exercise bike for 5-10 minutes) before performing these exercises.

Using a heel lift or a shoe with a moderate heel can help reduce the stress on the tendon.

MISCELLANY

In Greek mythology Achilles was dipped into the River Styx by his mother Thetis to coat his body with a shield of protection. Thetis grasped Achilles by the heel (on the eponymous tendon) when she dipped him, leaving that one area not washed by the river, and in turn unprotected. From that comes the term "Achilles heel," connoting a person's area of vulnerability.

KEY TERMS

Achilles tendonitis; insertional Achilles tendonitis; non-insertional Achilles tendonitis; Haglund's deformity; retrocalcaneal bursitis;

SKILLS

Bedside skills for the diagnosis of disorders of the Achilles include the ability to take a detailed but focused history and perform a thorough musculoskeletal examination.

CHAPTER 9.

ARTHROSIS OF THE ANKLE AND HINDFOOT

DESCRIPTION

Ankle arthrosis most commonly occurs after a major traumatic ankle injury. A pilon fracture may cause arthrosis of the tibiotalar (ankle) joint; a depressed calcaneal fracture can cause subtalar arthritis. Arthrosis is also seen after less severe injuries, especially if those injuries cause malalignment. Unlike the knee and hip, the ankle joint is a relatively uncommon site for the development of primary osteoarthritis. Arthrosis of the ankle is also treated with methods that would not be used in the knee or hip, as loss of motion to limit pain is better tolerated in the ankle and hindfoot. Thus, bracing and (in more extreme cases) surgical fusion is a commonly used method of treatment though surgical methods to restore small cartilage defects or to preserve motion through joint replacement are also used.

STRUCTURE AND FUNCTION

The ankle joint (talocrural or tibiotalar joint) is formed between the distal tibia and fibula and proximal talus (Figure 1). The superior talar dome has three articulating surfaces – medial, central, and lateral – that articulate with the medial malleolus, tibial plafond, and lateral malleolus, respectively. These articulations provide bony stability to the ankle joint when it is in a neutral or dorsiflexed position. In plantarflexion, the ankle joint has considerably less bony contact, and in that position relies more on the surrounding ligaments to provide stability.

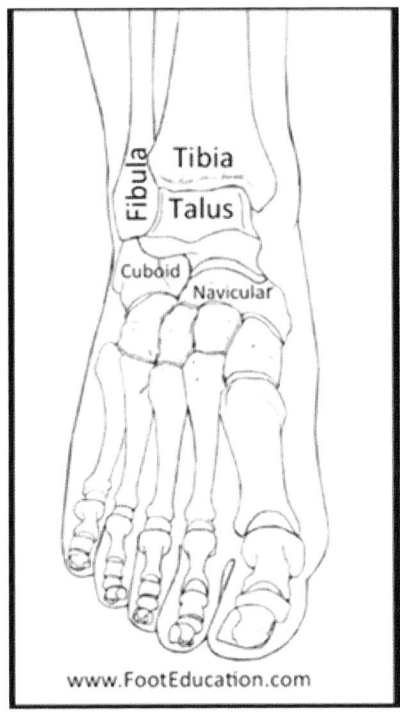

Figure 1: Ankle Bony Anatomy – Anterior View

The hindfoot consists of the calcaneus and talus (Figure 2). The inferior aspect of the talus articulates with the calcaneus inferiorly, forming the subtalar joint. The subtalar joint facilitates inversion and eversion of the foot.

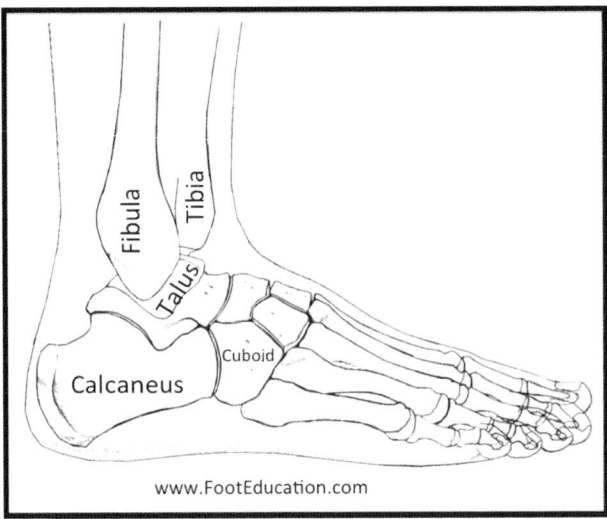

Figure 2: Ankle and Hindfoot Bony Anatomy – Lateral View

The talus is mostly covered by articular cartilage and has no muscular attachments, leaving little bone for vascular penetration. This lack of vascularity predisposes the talus to slow healing and avascular necrosis.

PATHOPHYSIOLOGY OF OSTEOARTHRITIS

The ankle joint surfaces are highly conforming, that is the surfaces have broad areas of contact. This allows the forces of weight-bearing to be spread out over a maximally large area and in turn minimizes focal joint pressure (Figure 3).

Injuries that damage the articular surfaces can decrease or change contact area, leading to high pressure in certain spots and predisposing the joint to further damage and arthrosis. The hallmark of osteoarthritis is the loss of articular cartilage. Major injury in the ankle will often start the process of osteoarthritis beginning with the breakdown of the joint surface and irritation of the synovium. Thereafter, there is impairment of chondrocyte function and sclerosis of the bone. In the final phase, there is overt disorganization and degeneration. Specifically, when the smooth articular cartilage is damaged, it becomes rough. Friction against the rough surface creates cartilage particles. The synovium absorbs these particles and may undergo a chronic low-grade inflammatory response, producing enzymes that cause further damage. In severe osteoarthritis (Figures 4 & 5), erosion of the articular surface can expose subchondral bone, allowing synovial fluid to enter the cancellous bone causing cysts. The subchondral bone may also thicken due to focal loading forming sclerotic bone. In addition, the inflammation of the joint present in arthritis may contribute to the formation of osteophytes (bone spurs) around the outside of the joint.

Osteoarthritis of the ankle and hindfoot is generally post-traumatic. Primary arthritis of the ankle, in contrast to the knee and hip, is rare.

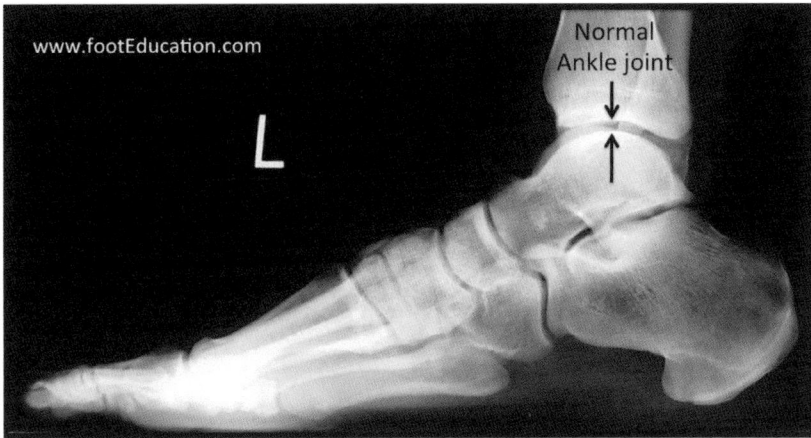

Figure 3: Normal ankle joint (Weight-bearing lateral x-ray).

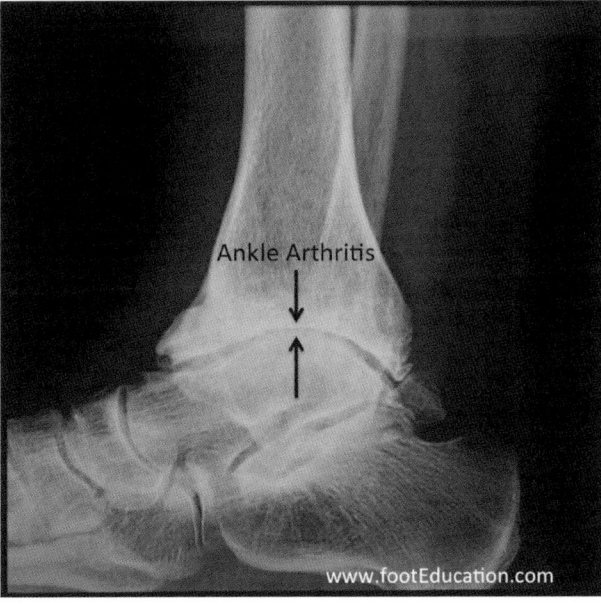

Figure 4: X-ray of severe ankle arthritis. Note joint space narrowing at the tibiotalar (ankle or talocrural) joint and anterior bone spur (osteophyte).

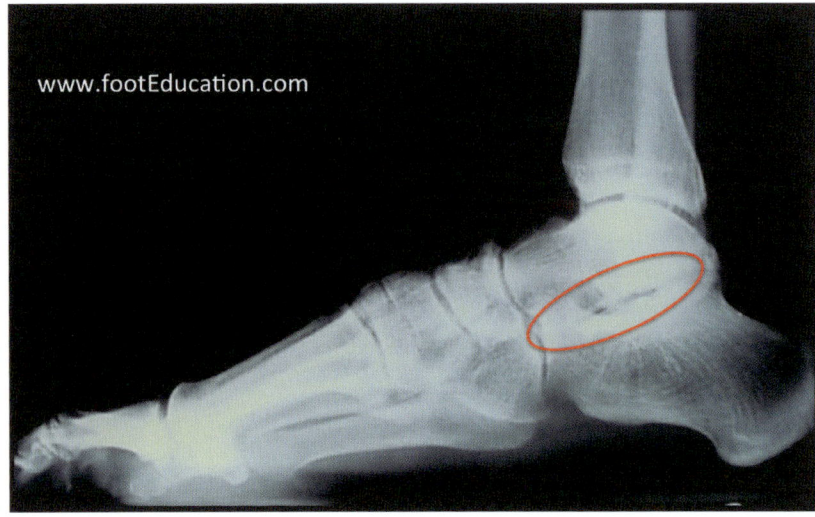

Figure 5: X-ray of subtalar arthritis. Note joint space narrowing at subtalar joint.

Osteochondral lesions of the talus can be thought of as a form of focal arthrosis: there is focal cartilage (and possibly bone) damage involving a relatively small portion of the ankle joint (Figure 6), while the remainder of the ankle joint is usually normal. Osteochondral lesions of the talus are also typically caused by trauma to the ankle. Usually it is more minor compressive and rotational forces that shear the cartilage and impact the underlying subchondral bone leading to edema (localized swelling) within the bone. Osteochondral lesions (OCL) of the talus can involve: cartilage only; cartilage and bone; subchondral bone with intact cartilage where there is solely edema of the bone; or where there is bone loss replaced with fluid in the form of a cyst underneath the cartilage. OCLs are typically classified according to whether they are stable/unstable and whether they are displaced or undisplaced.

Virtually all lateral talar OCLs (>90%) are due to trauma compared to roughly 60% of medial lesions. Lesions not caused by trauma may be caused by chronic overload to the foot, repeated microtrauma, avascular necrosis, or congenital factors.

Osteochondral lesions of the talus have poor healing due to the general avascularity of articular cartilage but also the tenuous vascular supply of the talus itself. Though OCLs do not typically heal, they also stay relatively stable over time and very rarely progress to arthritis that encompasses the whole joint.

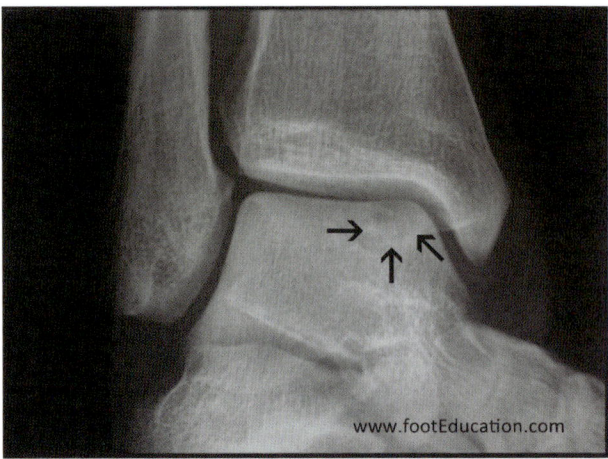

Figure 6: X-ray of medial osteochondral lesion of the talus.

PATIENT PRESENTATION

Patient presentation will vary depending on the type and location of arthrosis. In general, patients with hindfoot arthritis will present with pain, stiffness, and swelling. Symptoms are often exacerbated by activity and relieved with rest. It is important to determine the exact nature, location, duration, and progression of symptoms to narrow down the type of arthrosis and structures affected.

Localizing the area of maximal discomfort can narrow the differential. In the case of ankle osteoarthritis, pain is often on the anterior aspect of the ankle joint in a bandlike pattern along the tibiotalar joint. In subtalar arthritis, the pain is often localized to the lateral hindfoot, often underneath the fibula in the sinus tarsi, though sometimes the pain radiates medially as well. Patients with talar lesions often complain of localized ankle pain on either the medial or lateral sides of the ankle.

Identifying aggravating and alleviating factors can also help to identify the location of the arthritis. Pain with plantarflexion can indicate a posterior lesion of the talus, while dorsiflexion may aggravate an anterior lesion. If bone spurs are present impingement may occur with resulting pain as the bone spurs come into contact. Some patients may in fact wear high-top boots or shoes after they discover that these shoes alleviate symptoms by preventing excess dorsiflexion. Subtalar arthritis is commonly aggravated by walking on uneven ground because inversion/eversion occurs primarily at the subtalar joint.

Crepitus, catching, locking, grinding or the sensation of a loose body should increase your suspicion for an OLT with an unstable fragment. However, some patients with OLTs are asymptomatic and with the OCL being identified as an incidental finding on an MRI for another problem.

HISTORY

Patients with ankle or hindfoot arthrosis frequently describe a history of trauma to the joint (ankle fracture, tibia fracture, recurrent ankle sprains, etc.). This trauma may have been many years in the past. It is important to determine the type of injury – fracture or sprain – and the structures involved. A history of ankle inversion injury that doesn't improve with conservative treatment should heighten the examiner's suspicion for a persistent cartilage injury.

In patients in whom a history of trauma is not recalled, asking about personal history or family history of inflammatory arthritis (ex. rheumatoid arthritis) is important, though inflammatory arthritis normally presents elsewhere before affecting the ankle.

PHYSICAL EXAM

When evaluating a patient, check the alignment of the lower extremity – including the alignment of the knees and the hindfoot.

Determine the motion of the ankle and hindfoot joints by assessing ankle dorsiflexion and plantarflexion – and hindfoot inversion and eversion.

Assess for ankle stability using an anterior drawer test and a talar tilt test.

Other physical exam findings may include a joint effusion, tenderness to palpation over medial and/or lateral joint lines, decreased strength or calf atrophy from relative disuse.

Subtalar arthritis will tend to have hindfoot swelling, tenderness within the tarsal sinus, pain with inversion/eversion, and limited ROM at the subtalar joint. As always, perform a detailed neurovascular exam to look for weakness, loss of sensation, and decreased or absence of distal pulses.

When performing a physical examination, it is always important to look at both feet and ankles so that a normal baseline may be established for a patient.

OBJECTIVE EVIDENCE

Radiographic imaging is used to confirm a clinical diagnosis of arthrosis and often establishes the definitive diagnosis of arthritis. Weight-bearing anterior-posterior, lateral, and mortise/oblique views of the ankle and foot are required. Two additional views can also be used to evaluate the subtalar joint:

Broden's view (Figure 7): Foot internally rotated 45 degrees. X-ray angled 10-40 degrees cephalad. Used to evaluate the posterior subtalar facet.

Canale view (Figure 8): Foot pronated 15 degrees. X-ray aimed 75 degrees from horizontal on AP view. Used to evaluate the tarsal sinus.

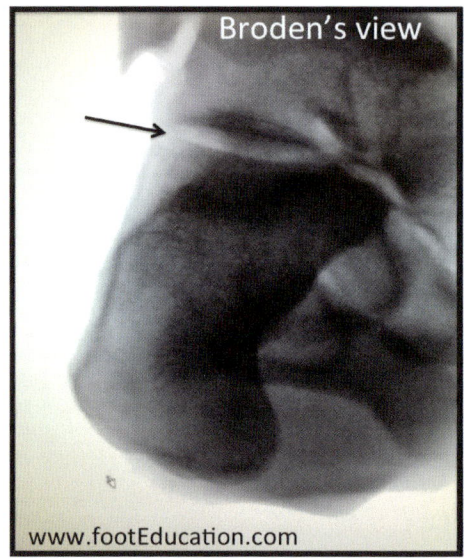

Figure 7: Broden's View highlighting the posterior facet of the subtalar joint

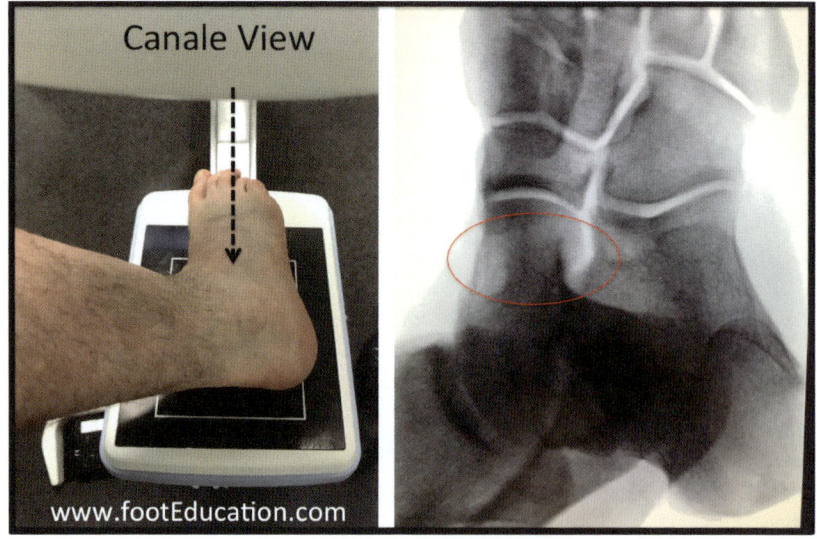

Figure 8: Canale View identifying the talar neck and sinus tarsi

Plain x-rays may demonstrate one or more of the four cardinal signs of arthritis:

1. Narrowing of the joint space,
2. Bone spurs (osteophytes),

3. Subchondral cysts, and
4. Bone whitening (subchondral sclerosis).

Radiographic imaging will not catch a purely cartilage injury or underlying bone edema. In these cases, if arthrosis is suspected but not visualized on x-ray, other imaging modalities (CT or MRI) are necessary to visualize the lesion. These modalities may also help determine if there is another source of pain (e.g., posterior tibial tendonitis, peroneal tendonitis, etc.).

A CT scan will provide a 3 dimensional view of the hindfoot and is generally used when trying to better visualize the 3 dimensional bony structure. CT scans can show subchondral cysts and joint space narrowing which are the hallmarks of arthritis and can help to visualize the subtalar joint that may not be visualized well on plain radiographs. It can also demonstrate the cystic change underneath an OCL.

MRI is a powerful tool because it can assess concomitant soft tissue pathology and chondral lesions with great accuracy (Figures 9). However, an MRI should only be ordered when there is a specific clinical question that needs to be answered (ex. "Does this patient have a OLT that is not seen on plain x-rays?") AND the answer to that question will change your management (ex. "Given this patient's symptoms if he/she has a large OLT on MRI, I will recommend surgery").

An MRI is rarely used in the diagnosis or treatment of ankle osteoarthritis, but it is more useful when focal talar lesions are suspected. MRI is the most sensitive tool for diagnosing these lesions because of its ability to detect bone bruising, cartilage damage, or fluid surrounding the lesions

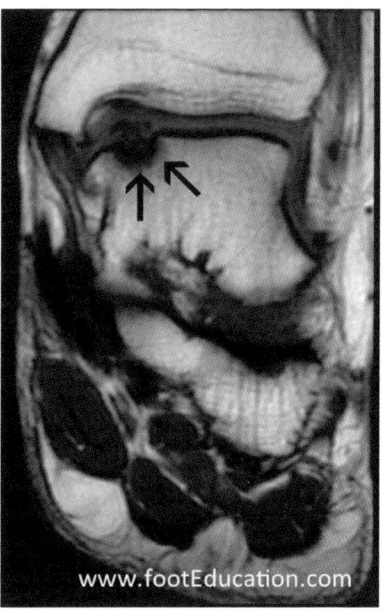

Figure 9: MRI of medial Osteochondral Lesion of the Talus (OLT).

Laboratory tests are generally not useful in diagnosing primary arthrosis but can be used to exclude other conditions such as rheumatoid arthritis and gout (See below).

A diagnostic injection of local anesthetic into the ankle or subtalar joint can also help confirm pain as originating from the ankle or subtalar arthritis. For example, if the pain is relieved for a few hours with an injection into the subtalar joint it suggests that the pain is likely originating from that joint. If the pain is not relieved, then other sources of pathology may need to be explored.

EPIDEMIOLOGY

Osteoarthritis of the ankle and hindfoot is less common than in other limb joints, partly because primary osteoarthritis of the foot and ankle is rare compared to the knee and hip. In a study by Saltzman et al (PMID: 16089071), of 639 patients with ankle arthritis, 70% were post-traumatic, 12% were rheumatoid in nature, and only 7% were idiopathic primary osteoarthritis. Loss of function and disability (limited walking ability, chronic pain, lower limb instability) are long-term consequences of ankle and hindfoot arthrosis.

DIFFERENTIAL DIAGNOSIS

Many conditions can present like ankle and hindfoot arthrosis. Injuries to the ankle ligaments, tendons and nerves as well as infections or masses may also cause pain in the ankle and should be differentiated from arthrosis of the ankle. Physical examination, imaging studies, and diagnostic injections can be helpful in narrowing the differential diagnosis.

Once arthrosis has been established the cause of arthritis should also be established as it may help direct the types of treatment offered.

Before deciding on a diagnosis of arthrosis, it is necessary to rule out the possibility of inflammatory arthritic conditions like rheumatoid arthritis, gout, as well as infectious arthritis. Obtaining a personal and family history of arthritis will help to narrow the differential. Lab tests like CBC, ESR, CRP, and immunohistochemistry can also help to identify inflammatory arthritic conditions. In cases where inflammatory or infectious arthritis is suspected, the most effective method for establishing a definitive diagnosis is made using a sample of synovial fluid attained through aspiration of the joint.

Avascular necrosis (also known as osteonecrosis) may present with symptoms typical of arthrosis before overt joint destruction is seen. It is most commonly associated with prolonged use of steroids (such as for people with asthma or other inflammatory conditions) or other medications.

TREATMENT OPTIONS AND OUTCOMES

Non-operative treatment

Non-operative treatment is usually indicated for patients with mild to moderate arthrosis but may be helpful for patients with any stage of arthritis. It normally involves a variety of treatments including: oral non-steroidal anti-inflammatory drugs and/or analgesics, physical therapy, and ankle stabilization (ex. ankle bracing). General exercise and activity modification can also help to prevent pain and progression of symptoms. In moderate-severe cases, intra-articular corticosteroid injection may be necessary to provide short-term pain relief.

Physical therapy is an important aspect of non-operative care early in the course of treatment, to maintain range of motion, strength, and proprioception and thereby decrease the likelihood of leg atrophy over time. Exercise that is relatively non-weight bearing (ex. swimming or cycling) may help maintain an ideal body weight because a high BMI can lead to excessive force on the affected joints.

Ankle support is an important aspect of non-operative care that can minimize painful joint motion and relieve pressure points. There are many ankle support options ranging from simple over-the-counter shoewear modification to ankle braces to custom-molded ankle-foot orthoses (AFOs).

Operative treatment

Operative treatment may be indicated in patients with severe osteoarthritis or when conservative treatment has failed. Several different surgical options exist for the treatment of osteoarthritis.

Arthroscopy: Arthroscopic procedures include synovectomy, debridement, loose body removal, excision of bone spurs, and chondroplasty. The effectiveness of ankle arthroscopy in the treatment of arthritis has not been assessed in randomized controlled trial. However, for patients with widespread arthritis it is unlikely to provide long-term relief. Arthroscopy may be helpful for patients with focal arthrosis with a talar OCL (See below).

Tibial osteotomy: Some cases of ankle arthritis stem from a tibial alignment deformity that leads to poor load distribution across the ankle joint. In these cases tibial osteotomy can correct alignment, and improve load distribution across the ankle joint. It is indicated in young patients with a varus or valgus deformity and mild to moderate arthritis caused by a tibial deformity.

Ankle arthrodesis (Figure 10): Ankle arthrodesis (tibiotalar fusion) is one of the most predictable means of relieving pain from severe ankle arthritis and can be highly effective at doing so. The fusion can be performed either open or arthroscopically to remove the remaining cartilage from the two sides of joint, with additional fixation with plates and/or screws to hold the bones until fusion is achieved. Fusion rates are similar between the two methods, about 80 to 90%, and patient factors such as deformity, vascular or skin compromise, and bone quality often dictate the method used. The major disadvantage of arthrodesis is that it sacrifices the plantarflexion and dorsiflexion movements of the ankle joint. The lack of ankle motion from fusion may be mildly impairing and may also accelerate arthrosis in the subtalar joint. In order to maximize the motion in surrounding joints following fusion, the ankle should be positioned in neutral dorsiflexion and slight hindfoot valgus (heel angled to the outside).

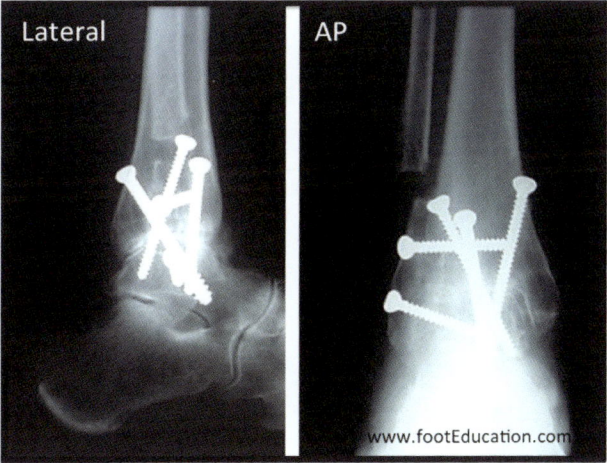

Figure 10: Ankle Arthrodesis (Ankle Fusion).

Total Ankle Arthroplasty (TAA): In this procedure, the surgeon replaces the damaged tibial plafond and talus with an artificial joint (Figure 11). It is ideal for a lightweight, sedentary, older patient with end-stage osteoarthritis who has minimal deformity, good range of motion, and a good soft tissue envelope. It has a similar ability to relieve pain as arthrodesis, but with the advantage of preserving motion and possibly relieving stress on adjacent joints. The major disadvantage of ankle joint replacement is that it is mechanical, and will eventually wear out and possibly need a revision replacement. This tends to happen more quickly than in either hip or knee replacements, though recent studies have shown a successful ankle implant retention rate approaching 85-90% at 8-10 years.

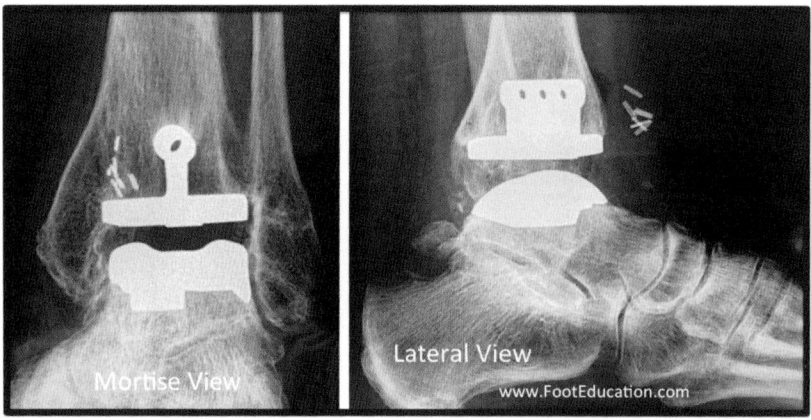

Figure 11: Total Ankle Arthroplasty

<u>Subtalar arthrodesis</u>: Fusion of the subtalar joint (Figure 12) is the best treatment for subtalar arthritis that has failed non-operative treatment. This procedure involves removing the joint cartilage and subchondral bone and attaching the two sides of the subtalar joint with screws or staples. If the two surfaces of the joint do not fully oppose each other then bone graft, either autograft or allograft may be used to fill the void and promote fusion. Again, the tradeoff inherent in any fusion procedure (loss of pain at the price of loss of motion) applies here as well. The procedure can be extended to include the talo-navicular and calcaneo-cubiod joints This is called a "triple arthrodesis." It is most commonly used to correct deformity within the hindfoot.

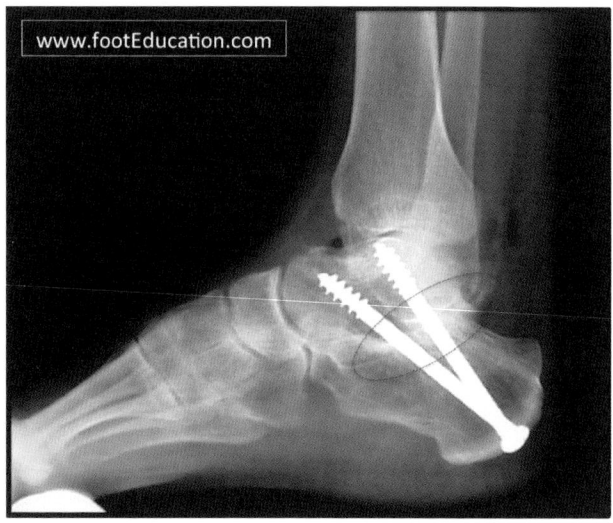

Figure 12: X-ray of Subtalar Arthrodesis (Subtalar Fusion).

<u>Debridement and microfracture</u>: This is the most common approach for treating small (<1.5cm in diameter) talar OCLS. The unstable cartilage is arthroscopically trimmed back and then the bony base is cracked with a pick or drill ("microfractured") to stimulate bleeding and subsequent formation of a fibrin clot. The fibrin clot that fills the defect undergoes transformation into fibrocartilage (type I cartilage). It is successful in about 90% of cases in which the OLT lesion is less than <15mm. If the articular surface is intact, yet there is a lesion right below it, drilling the talus from distal to proximal, up to, but not through, the articular surface (so called "retrograde drilling") may be used.

<u>Transplantation of osteochondral tissue</u>: Several transplantation techniques exist to replace lost articular cartilage including osteochondral autograft or allograft transplantation (OATS) and autologous chondrocyte implantation (ACI). These procedures are usually reserved for lesions that have failed debridement and micro fracture, or for larger lesions.

During the OATS procedures, cylinders of cartilage and underlying bone are harvested from the femoral condyle or trochlea and placed within the lesion (not unlike hair plugs). The ACI procedure comprises harvesting autologous chondrocytes, expanding them in a laboratory culture and then re-implanting this larger mass of cells into the lesion, covered by a periosteal patch or collagen matrix.

RISK FACTORS AND PREVENTION

Since ankle and hindfoot arthrosis are normally caused by trauma, risk factors are the same as those for ankle and hindfoot injuries including fractures, recurrent ankle sprains, and malalignment. Sports like soccer, football, and basketball have an increased risk of these injuries and therefore have an increased risk of arthrosis.

Some congenital deformities of the foot (e.g. clubfoot) place the patient at increased risk for ankle and hindfoot arthrosis.

MISCELLANY

Aviator's astragalus is an old term referring to a displaced talar neck fracture with associated compression fractures of the talus – a pattern of injury seen in World War I aviators who crashed their planes. This term is now only a historical curiosity. These fractures, if displaced have a high rate of osteonecrosis which often leads to either tibiotalar or subtalar arthritis or both.

KEY TERMS

Osteoarthritis, Ankle arthritis, subtalar arthritis, Osteochondritis dissecans, Talar osteochondral lesions, Loose body, Talar dome lesion, Ankle arthrodesis, Ankle arthroplasty, Aviator's astragalus

SKILLS

Examine the ankle and hindfoot for tenderness, deformity, and instability. Differentiate ankle and hindfoot arthrosis from other types of arthritis based on history, physical exam, imaging, and other diagnostic testing. Localize arthrosis to the talocrural or subtalar joint.

CHAPTER 10.

TARSAL TUNNEL SYNDROME

DESCRIPTION

Tarsal tunnel syndrome is a condition that causes pain in the foot due to traction and compression of the tibial nerve within the tarsal tunnel. The tarsal tunnel is located in the ankle behind the medial malleolus, superficial to the bones (calcaneus and talus) and covered by the flexor retinaculum. When the posterior tibial nerve is irritated presenting symptoms include pain, numbness and paresthesias. Tarsal tunnel syndrome can be caused by space occupying lesions (such as a ganglion cyst); more commonly it is caused by deformities of the foot and ankle that stretch the nerve and decrease the volume of the tarsal tunnel.

STRUCTURE AND FUNCTION

The tarsal tunnel is the space located posterior and inferior to the medial malleolus; medial to the calcaneus and talus, and deep to the flexor retinaculum. The contents of the tarsal tunnel, from anterior to posterior, include the tibialis posterior tendon, the flexor digitorum longus tendon, the posterior tibial artery, tibial nerve, and flexor hallucis longus (Figure 1). The tibial nerve divides within the tarsal tunnel into the calcaneal nerve coursing towards the heel and the medial and lateral plantar nerves which supply the bottom of the foot.

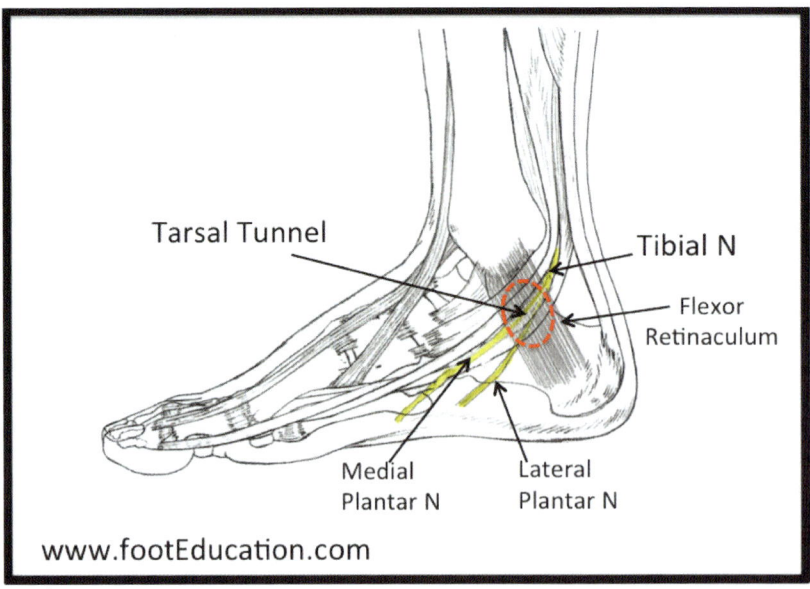

Figure 1: Tarsal Tunnel Anatomy

The flexor retinaculum – also known as the laciniate ligament – covering the tunnel ensures that the contents of the tunnel remain within it, but may be a source of abnormal compression if the anatomy is disturbed.

Tarsal tunnel syndrome is thought to be caused by repetitive traction on the nerve leading to scarring. In this sense the etiology of the condition is different than carpal tunnel in the wrist which is primarily a compression-related phenomenon. However, extrinsic compression from a bone spur, ganglion, or synovial proliferation from a tendon disorder, although much less common, may also cause tarsal tunnel syndrome.

As pressure increases with the tarsal tunnel, blood flow decreases and the nerve becomes ischemic. Malfunction of the nerve, in turn, yield the presenting symptoms of tingling and numbness.

PATIENT PRESENTATION

Patients with tarsal tunnel syndrome typically complain of numbness in the foot radiating to the big toe and the first 3 toes, pain, burning, electrical sensations, and tingling over the base of the foot and the heel. A broader area of symptoms suggests either nerve entrapment proximal to the tarsal tunnel, or a generalized neuropathy.

Standing, especially in patients with associated flatfoot deformities, causes increased traction and compression on the nerve within the tarsal tunnel. As a result, patients may report that prolonged standing and walking makes their symptoms worse.

Compression of the tibial artery within the tarsal tunnel may cause ischemia to the intrinsic muscles of the foot with painful cramping accordingly.

OBJECTIVE EVIDENCE

On physical examination, patients will often have a flat foot.

Palpation over the tarsal tunnel will produce localized pain (tenderness) as well as radiating pain into the sole of the foot (Figure 2). This latter sensation with percussion of the nerve is called a "Tinel's sign," though this is not a true objective sign but a vocalized subjective symptom. Sensory examination of the foot may reveal some decreased sensation on the sole of the foot, although in most patients this is not the case.

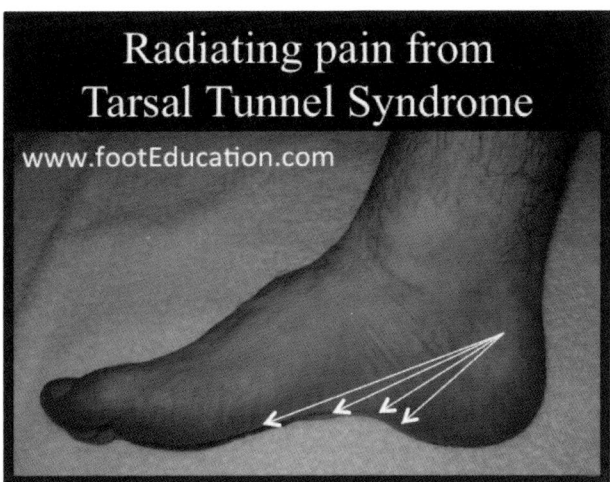

Figure 2: Location of Pain in Tarsal Tunnel Syndrome

Muscle atrophy and claw-toe deformities suggest chronic compression.

Nerve conduction studies will often show a decrease in conduction velocity in the tibial nerve precisely as it courses under the flexor retinaculum.

Weight-bearing x-rays of the foot should be assessed to exclude fractures and bone spurs, as well as malalignment (for example, hindfoot varus or valgus) that can alter the geometry of the tarsal tunnel.

CT scans, ultrasound or MRI might be needed to rule out space-occupying lesions within the tarsal tunnel (Figure 3). These include ganglions, lipomas, or (rarely) accessory muscles. Detection of a mass on imaging studies is uncommon, but critical to rule out. When a space-occupying lesion is present the patient is unlikely to improve clinically until the mass is removed. By contrast, without a mass, surgery is rarely indicated.

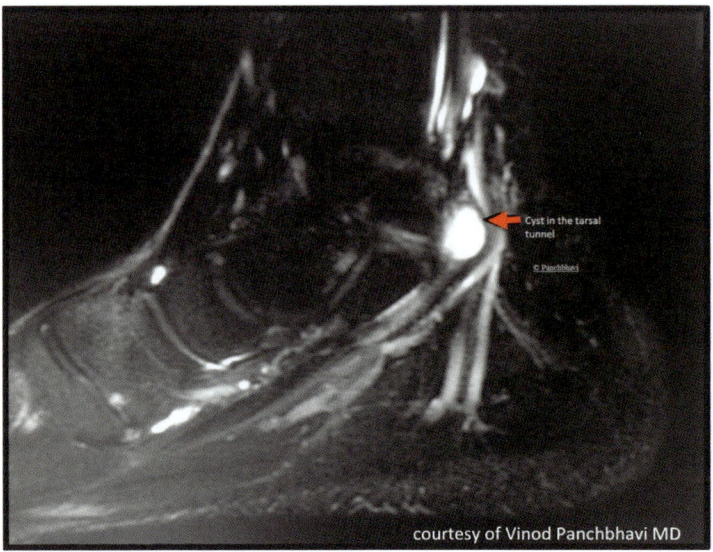

Figure 3: MRI showing a fluid-filled ganglion that is compressing the tibial nerve. (courtesy of Vinod Panchbhavi MD)

EPIDEMIOLOGY

The National Institutes of Health's website on rare diseases says, "The incidence and prevalence of tarsal tunnel syndrome is unknown." (https://rarediseases.info.nih.gov/diseases/7733/tarsal-tunnel-syndrome). The very fact that tarsal tunnel syndrome is included by the NIH on its list of "rare" conditions means that it affects fewer than 200,000 people in the United States.

DIFFERENTIAL DIAGNOSIS

The differential diagnosis of tarsal tunnel syndrome can be considered to have two components. The first is the true differential diagnosis – that is, the list of conditions that may instead be responsible for a presentation similar to that of tarsal tunnel syndrome. Beyond that, once the diagnosis is established, there is a second differential diagnosis list to consider, namely, the other conditions that may be responsible for causing the tarsal tunnel syndrome itself.

In the first category, the main considerations are lumbar radiculopathy and peripheral neuropathy (most often caused by diabetes). A complex regional pain syndrome (formerly known as Reflex Sympathetic Dystrophy) could be responsible as well, though the findings in complex regional pain syndrome would almost certainly extend beyond the distribution of the tibial nerve.

Conditions that may be the cause of tarsal tunnel syndrome include trauma (fracture fragments causing compression or ligament injury causing instability and traction on the nerve); space-occupying lesions such as ganglion cyst, benign tumors, swollen tendons or varicose veins; ankle deformities such as pes planus (flat foot).

In addition, there are associated conditions that are commonly found in patients with tarsal tunnel syndrome owing to a similar etiology. Acquired adult flatfoot deformity (posterior tibial tenosynovitis) and plantar fasciitis tend to occur in patients with flatfeet due to repetitive traction loading of these structures. Similar traction forces often produce tarsal tunnel like symptoms.

RED FLAGS

There are no true "red flags" with tarsal tunnel syndrome, though the presentation of tarsal tunnel syndrome-like complaints may be the first clue of an otherwise undetected diagnosis of diabetes, peripheral artery disease or disc herniation/spinal stenosis.

TREATMENT OPTIONS AND OUTCOMES

If the patient has confirmed tarsal tunnel syndrome caused by a space-occupying lesion, that offending structure should be removed. Beyond that, the vast majority of patients with tarsal tunnel syndrome can (and should) be treated non-operatively. Only with a prolonged failure of non-operative treatment in a patient with positive nerve conduction studies and severe symptoms should surgical release be considered.

The primary non-operative treatment approach to treating tarsal tunnel syndrome is to attempt to decrease the repetitive traction injury across the nerve and the other structures in this area of the foot. In this regard, treatment is quite similar to that for acquired adult flatfoot deformity and plantar fasciitis.

Comfort shoes designed to disperse the force more evenly across the foot can be very helpful. Weight loss should be recommended to patients who need it.

A prefabricated orthotic with a supportive arch will help to disperse the force more evenly across the foot may also be helpful.

Physical therapy including exercises designed to stretch the calf muscle and thereby indirectly decrease the load through this area of the foot may also be helpful.

Limiting walking can reduce symptoms but may impede weight loss (and be impractical for other reasons). Advice to limit standing, an activity which can produce symptoms with fewer health benefits than those involving motion, may be more apt.

Corticosteroid injections may help to decrease the swelling around the nerve in the short and intermediate term. However, it is unclear what effect they have in the long term. In addition it is possible to injure the nerve during the injection process.

Operative treatment can be considered in rare cases. Primary resection of space-occupying lesions causing isolated tarsal tunnel syndrome can relieve symptoms reliably, provided that the nerve is neither scarred nor damaged prior to surgery. Beyond that, operative treatment includes tarsal tunnel release and other procedures to correct deformity causing compression may be used.

Tarsal tunnel release comprises release of the flexor retinaculum and neurolysis of the tibial nerve and its branches. The latter includes removal of scar tissue, if any, as well as fascial releases. Problems with a tarsal tunnel release include that the procedure does not address the traction on the structures within the tarsal tunnel (often the primary issue) and that additional scar tissue often reforms in the post-surgical period due to the operative procedure.

There is limited evidence that surgery is effective. One study in the Journal of Bone and Joint Surgery [https://www.ncbi.nlm.nih.gov/pubmed/8056802] reported a 38% incidence of patients "clearly dissatisfied with the result and had no long-term relief of the pain." Complications were seen in 13% of patients as well, including three wound infections.

RISK FACTORS AND PREVENTION

Tarsal tunnel syndrome is known to affect individuals that stand a lot. Strenuous activities involving repetitive eversion, inversion, and plantarflexion at high velocities can produce the symptoms of tarsal tunnel syndrome. Patients with underlying flatfoot deformities are more likely to have associated tarsal tunnel symptoms.

Obesity is a double risk factor in that weight alone can cause mechanical overload, but it is also associated with diabetes (which causes a neuropathy that may make the nerve less tolerant of even mild compression).

Rheumatoid arthritis, hypothyroidism and gout are thought to be associated with tarsal tunnel syndrome.

MISCELLANY

The anterior to posterior arrangement of the structures coursing through the tarsal tunnel (namely: the <u>T</u>ibialis posterior tendon, the flexor <u>D</u>igitorum longus tendon, the posterior tibial <u>A</u>rtery and <u>V</u>ein, the tibial <u>N</u>erve, and the flexor <u>H</u>allucis longus tendon) can be recalled with this mnemonic: "<u>T</u>om, <u>D</u>ick, <u>A</u>nd <u>V</u>ery <u>N</u>ervous <u>H</u>arry."

KEY TERMS

Tarsal tunnel, posterior tibial nerve, pes planus, plantar fasciitis, tarsal tunnel release

SKILLS

Perform a comprehensive history and physical that can identify tarsal tunnel syndrome as well as rival conditions on the differential diagnosis list. Recognize the deformities of the foot and ankle that may place undue traction on the posterior tibial nerve.

CHAPTER 11.

RHEUMATOID DISORDERS OF THE FOOT AND ANKLE

DESCRIPTION

Rheumatoid arthritis (RA) is an autoimmune chronic inflammatory condition where the body's immune system attacks the joints and causes inflammation of the joint lining (synovium). Typically RA is a symmetrical polyarthritis, affecting multiple small joints of the hands and feet bilaterally, and more than 90% of RA patients develop symptoms in the foot and ankle over time.

STRUCTURE AND FUNCTION

Diarthrodial joints, which include the type found between the bones of the feet, are lined by the synovium. The synovium produces a synovial fluid to lubricate the joint, reduce friction, and help absorb shock. Normal synovial tissue has thin monolayer of cells containing monocyte-derived cells that remove debris, cells that produce hyaluronic acid, and fibroblasts that produce lubricin.

Pathophysiology of rheumatoid arthritis

Rheumatoid arthritis is an inflammatory disease of the synovium, often affecting the small joints of the hands and feet (MTP, PIP, DIP joints). The etiology of RA is likely an interplay of genetics, environmental triggers, and immune response leading to an autoimmune attack on the body's own tissue. In brief, the synovial membrane is infiltrated by macrophages, lymphocytes, plasma cells, and granulocytes. Macrophages secrete matrix metalloproteinases and other proteolytic enzymes that damage the synovial tissue. Plasma cells release rheumatoid factor (RF) and other immunoglobulins that perpetuate the inflammatory response.

PATIENT PRESENTATION

A typical patient will likely be female, aged 40 to 60 presenting with pain, stiffness, swelling, and limited range of motion in the joints, prototypically those of the wrists and hands. Initial involvement in the feet occurs in 15% of cases. The stiffness seen in RA is most often worst in the morning, and may last one or two hours. The morning stiffness is due to a build-up of extracellular fluid in and around the joint. Other signs and symptoms are systemic and include loss of energy and appetite, dry eyes and fever. A dry mouth and firm lumps beneath the skin (so-called rheumatoid nodules) may also be seen.

In the lower extremity, RA more commonly affects the forefoot; the midtarsal joints are next most likely to be involved. The forefoot is involved twice as often as the hindfoot.

The changes that occur to the forefoot in patients with RA span a combination of bunions, claw toes, and metatarsalgia. These changes occur because the inflamed synovium causes the associated joint capsule to become lax leading to deformity or even dislocation of the involved joint. Hallux valgus can be quite severe and the big toe commonly crosses over the second toe. Calluses can also form on the ball of the foot when midfoot bones are pushed down from joint dislocations in the toes (MTP joints). As a result, callosities and even ulcers on the plantar forefoot can form from the abnormal pressure.

In the midfoot, RA can weaken the ligaments that support the midfoot causing collapse of the arch. Bony prominences can appear on the arch. Rupture of the tibialis posterior tendon can occur, and if it does, the talonavicular joint and subtalar joints sublux and the hindfoot drifts into valgus, leading to midfoot hyperpronation and a marked acquired adult flatfoot deformity (fallen arch).

OBJECTIVE EVIDENCE

Radiographs may show soft tissue swelling, subchondral bone erosions, osteopenia, joint space narrowing, bony destruction, and the classic finding of peri-articular erosions. Osteopenia starts in the metaphyseal region underlying collateral ligament attachments and becomes more generalized as the disease progresses. Inflamed synovium can wear away the bone at the point where the collateral ligaments attach creating characteristic peri-articular erosions (Figure 1). Cartilage destruction occurs when the inflamed synovium extends into the joint itself growing on top of the cartilage (pannus). This leads to destruction of the cartilage over time and narrowing of the joint on plain x-rays. Mal-alignment, displacement, and ankylosis of the joint mark end-stage rheumatoid disease.

Synovial fluid: Aspiration and analysis of the synovial fluid is important for distinguishing RA from non-inflammatory and infectious arthrosis. The fluid in patients with RA will be sterile, with increased neutrophils and increased protein but decreased viscosity. Obtaining a fluid sample from small joints in the feet in early stages can be very difficult and not clinically practical in many cases.

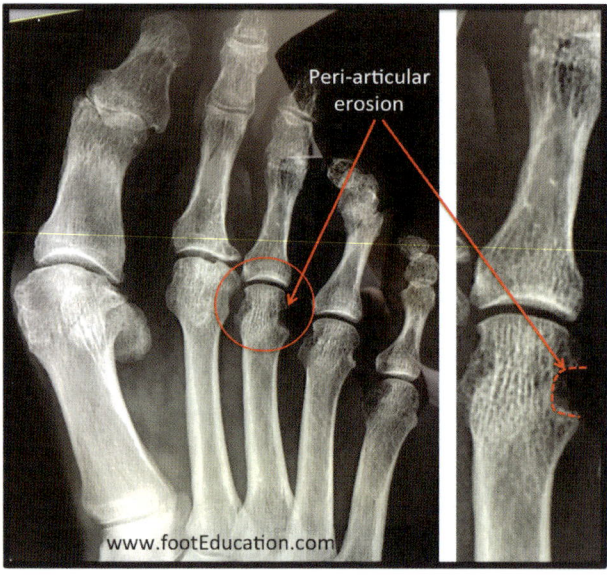

Figure 1: Radiograph showing Peri-articular Erosions

EPIDEMIOLOGY

RA is the most common of the inflammatory arthritides affecting about 1% of people, with female:male ratio of 3:1. The peak incidence is at age 50, and symptoms most commonly develop between age 40 to 60.

DIFFERENTIAL DIAGNOSIS

RA of the foot can present with findings that may suggest other conditions including:

- Crystal induced arthritis(gout/pseudogout): usually involves the knee, the metatarsal-phalangeal joint of the big toe, and the heel, and can be diagnosed with an aspiration of the joint fluid.
- Osteoarthritis: usually seen in older patients and affects weight-bearing joints asymmetrically. Pain worsens with prolonged use of the joint. Can be distinguished with x-rays.
- Systemic lupus erythematosus: characterized by the "butterfly rash" on the face, photosensitivity, joint pain in the hands and feet, and presence of antibodies against double-stranded DNA.
- Scleroderma: joint inflammation, compression syndromes (carpal tunnel is often an initial symptom of scleroderma).
- Psoriatic arthritis: distinguished by nail and skin changes.
- Lyme disease: check patient's history of presence in endemic regions and order appropriate blood tests as necessary to diagnose.
- Reiter's syndrome(reactive arthritis): asymmetrically involves the heel, sacroiliac joints, and large joints of the leg. Also associated with urethritis, conjunctivitis, iritis and painless buccal ulcers.
- Ankylosing spondylitis: though this involves the spine, it's possible that RA-like symmetrical, small-joint polyarthritis might also occur in AS.
- Hepatitis C: may induce Rheumatoid factor auto-antibodies, and can cause RA-like symmetrical small-joint polyarthritis.
- Acute rheumatic fever: migratory pattern of joint involvement (usually asymmetric), with history of antecedent streptococcal infection.
- Gonococcal arthritis: migratory pattern involving tendons around ankles and wrists, with history of antecedent gonococcal infection.

RED FLAGS

RA can be systemic. Consider the diagnosis of RA as a red flag to prompt an evaluation of problems elsewhere. As a systemic disease RA can affect blood vessels, nerves, and tendons throughout the body. Patients with extra-articular manifestation are more likely to have a high RF titer, more severe disability, and increased mortality rate.

TREATMENT OPTIONS AND OUTCOMES

There is currently no cure for RA. Medical treatments focus on controlling the disease and preventing progressive loss of function of the joints. As many of the symptoms of RA stem from the resulting joint deformity or loss of articular cartilage, early aggressive treatment is very important.

NSAIDs and corticosteroids (oral or injections) are used to alleviate inflammation and vasculitis. There are now a series of disease modifying anti-rheumatic drugs (DMARDs) that slow progression and improve symptoms, function, and quality of life. Common DMARDs include Methotrexate and biologic agents such as etanercept, infliximab and adalimumab that offer a more specific approach by targeting the pro-inflammatory cytokine TNF.

In the case of flare-ups of the foot and ankle, considerable relief can be gained from the use of appropriate footwear and insoles. Stiff soled comfort shoes with a soft accommodative orthotic and a wide toe box can be very helpful in patients with RA. An orthotic and/or a rocker soled shoe can support RA involvement of the midfoot (arch) and ankle. Some patients may benefit from the use of ankle bracing or even use of a removable walking cast boot.

In cases of an acquired adult flatfoot deformity (collapse of the arch) secondary to an RA induced posterior tibial tendon dysfunction a surgical reconstruction may be indicated. When RA affects the posterior tibial tendon, early synovectomy of the tendon sheath relieves discomfort and can delay or prevent rupture. When posterior tibial tendon rupture has occurred, transfer of the flexor digitorum longus tendon to the distal posterior tibial tendon stump combined with a subtalar fusion or a medializing calcaneal osteotomy may be necessary.

Foot surgery in the RA patient needs to be tailored to the specific deformity. For example, talonavicular arthritis is common in RA patients. These patients often do well with a fusion of the talonavicular joint using a bone graft. This can alleviate the pain from this joint and provide the foot with a stable medial beam, thereby helping to prevent the calcaneus from taking a fixed valgus position.

If RA of the forefoot has severely progressed with dislocation of many of the MTP joints one option is the Hoffman procedure -a procedure that removes all of the metatarsal heads in the foot. The bony prominence of the metatarsal heads are removed shifting the weight-bearing surface to the bottom of the foot. This MTP joint sacrificing procedure should be performed only in advanced disease, as it is quite destructive and non-anatomic. This procedure is usually reserved for the lesser (2-5) MTP joints only and is often combined with arthrodesis (fusion) of the 1st MTP (big toe) joint (Clayton procedure).

Patient with significant RA involving the hindfoot will often develop marked pain and associated deformity. These patients may benefit from a triple arthrodesis. This procedure realigns and fuses the talonavicular, subtalar, and calcaneocuboid joints. Fusion allow the deformity to be corrected, improves stability of the hindfoot, and eliminates pain from the arthritic joints thereby allowing for easier weight-bearing. A potential complication is that other joints of the foot may develop arthritis over time as they will be subject to more stress after a triple arthrodesis.

RISK FACTORS AND PREVENTION

Risk factors include HLA-DR4 haplotype; female gender; smoking history; and periodontal disease. While alone it has not been associated with increased risk of developing RA, obesity has been linked to poorer prognosis and response to treatment modalities.

MISCELLANY

Synovium is partially derived from the word *ovum*, Latin for egg, because of the yolk-like consistency of synovial fluid.

KEY TERMS

Synovitis, morning stiffness, inflammatory arthritis, rheumatoid factor, ACPA, HLA-DR4, symmetrical polyarthritis, claw toes

SKILLS

Recognize RA and distinguish it from osteoarthritis. Analyze synovial fluid and distinguish inflammatory vs non-inflammatory, and infectious vs non-infectious arthritides. Assess joint damage in radiographs.

CHAPTER 12.

DIABETIC FOOT DISORDERS

DESCRIPTION

Diabetes is a medical condition characterized by many complications, including neuropathy and peripheral artery disease. Loss of sensation in neuropathy can lead to ulceration of the skin and accelerated degeneration of the joint (a condition known as Charcot arthropathy); and poor vascularity can impede healing.

PATHOLOGY AND PATHOPHYSIOLOGY

Neuropathy is the initiating event in the development of most diabetic foot ulcers and infections. However joint contractures, excess localized pressure and vascular disease also play a role in their formation. The development of peripheral neuropathy in individuals with diabetes is attributed to a complex interaction of glycosylated hemoglobin with arterioles of both central and peripheral nerves, leading to conduction defects in sensory, motor, and autonomic function.

Prolonged exposure to even low pressure over a bony prominence (as may be seen with ill-fitting shoes) can cause skin breakdown. In patients without neuropathy this pressure will cause pain, and the person will shift his or her weight to limit the pressure. With a loss of such protective sensation, loading continues to the point that the skin breaks down and an ulcer forms (Figure 1). Without adequate off-loading of the area, ulcers can worsen leading to a local infection, progression to osteomyelitis, and eventual amputation in some patients.

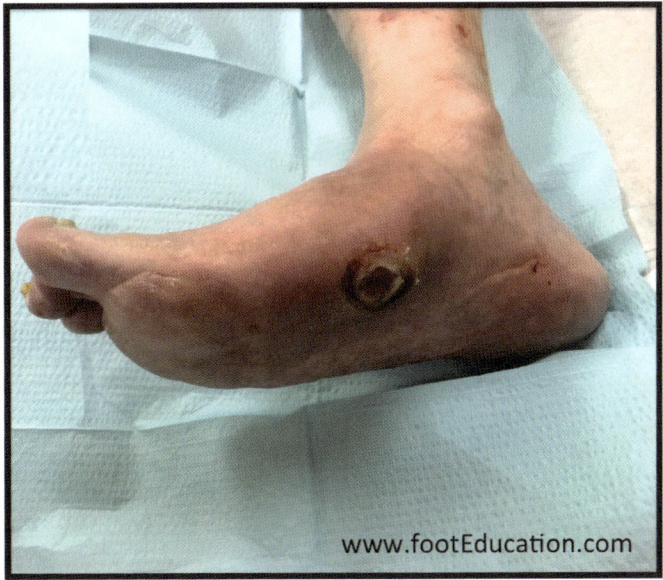

Figure 1: Diabetic Ulcer of plantar medial midfoot due to Charcot deformity

Charcot arthropathy is characterized by joint fragmentation and subluxation caused by continued repetitive stress to the foot and ankle in patients with peripheral neuropathy. The condition is named after Jean Marie Charcot (1825-1893) who described the collapse of the bones of the foot in patients who had loss of sensation in the feet from tertiary syphilis. The three commonly affected locations in the foot and ankle are the tarsal-metatarsal joints (midfoot), the transverse tarsal joint (hindfoot just in front of the ankle), and the ankle joint.

According to the *neurotraumatic theory*, Charcot arthropathy occurs as a result of cumulative mechanical trauma. This is usually unrecognized microtrauma due to neuropathy, but can also occur from major trauma such as bumping the foot or twisting an ankle. The *neurovascular theory* holds that an autonomic peripheral neuropathy creates increased blow flow that leads to increased bone resorption and ligamentous weakening, leading to joint destruction. In a simplified version of this theory, increased blood flow "washes out" structural calcium from the bone, leading to localized osteopenia and structurally inferior bone that ultimately collapses. (A more detailed version posits that proinflammatory cytokines such as IL-1 and TNF alpha activate the RANK (Receptor Activator of Nuclear Factor ϰ B) ligand pathway, causing up-regulation of NF-ϰB (nuclear factor kappa-light-chain-enhancer of activated B cells) which leads to increased osteoclastogenesis and osteolysis.) Most likely, a combination of both theories contributes to this condition.

PATIENT PRESENTATION

Diabetic Foot Ulceration

Patients with diabetic foot ulcers present commonly with swelling, discharge or a foul-smelling odor from the affected foot. The ulcer can be a source of pain but many times, the foot will be painless due to the loss of sensation to the area. Ulcerations are often found incidentally by the patient or primary caregiver.

Physical examination should be focused on the location of the ulcer as well as the depth. The size of the ulcer, perfusion, loss of sensation, signs of inflammation, the presence of gangrenous tissue, and signs of infection such as exudate or odor should also be noted. Loss of sensation can be documented by lack of ability to detect a 5.07 Semmes-Weinstein monofilament

Typically, ulcers will occur over a prominent area such as the metatarsal heads, although any area of the foot that is subject to a concentrated, repetitive force is at risk for developing a diabetic ulceration.

Diabetic Foot Charcot Arthropathy

Patients with Charcot arthropathy of the foot often present with unilateral swelling, redness, and increased skin temperature around the midfoot or ankle (Figure 2). Most patients present in their fifth or sixth decade and have peripheral neuropathy. Many are obese and have had diabetes for many years.

Charcot arthropathy can be painful. However classically, the patient presents with a swollen, warm, and erythematous painless foot. Charcot arthropathy is commonly mistaken for an infection (e.g., osteomyelitis) especially when there is an ulcer present. One strategy for differentiating an acute Charcot foot from infection is to elevate the foot several minutes. In Charcot, the erythema will resolve, while in infection it does not.

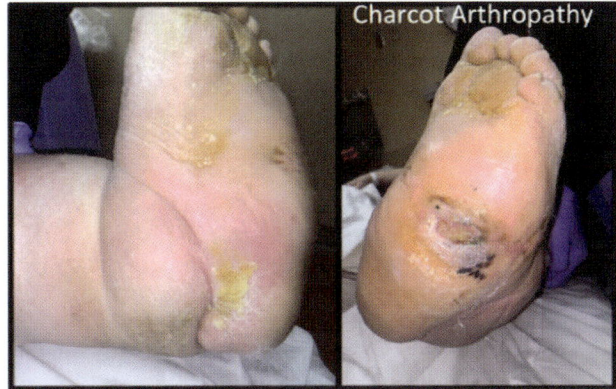

Figure 2: Severe Charcot Arthropathy. Patient with diabetes mellitus presented with a diffusely swollen, warm and non-tender left ankle and foot due to Charcot arthropathy (Image courtesy of Michael Swords MD)

OBJECTIVE EVIDENCE

Diabetic foot ulcers should be characterized objectively by location and severity. There are multiple classification systems to grade ulcers:

The *Wagner system* rates ulcers on a 0 to 6 scale, from "0: skin intact" to "6: ulcer with extensive foot gangrene."

The *Brodsky system* considers both the extent to the ulcer (superficial, deep and exposed bone) as well as the extent of ischemia.

The vascular status of the foot should also be assessed objectively, noting the skin color and temperature, the quality of capillary refill and presence or absence of palpable pulses. The ankle-brachial index (ABI), namely the ratio of the blood pressure in the ankle relative to that in the arm can be assessed in the clinic, though calcification of the vessels may produce a falsely normal result. Values of 1.0-1.4 is a normal ABI result. Whereas, an ABI value of <0.5 represents severe arteriole disease.

IMAGING STUDIES

In patients presenting with an ulcer, standard weight-bearing anteroposterior, lateral, and oblique radiographs of the affected foot should be obtained. Weight-bearing x-rays should be performed whenever possible. These films can detect deformities of the foot in general, as well as bone changes such as periosteal reaction, bone fragmentation, joint subluxations, lucencies or osteolysis (Figure 3).

MRI may be helpful to determine the extent of bony and soft-tissue disruption, but MRI cannot differentiate between Charcot arthropathy and osteomyelitis with high specificity. Occasionally, a bone scan is indicated, although very often the results of the bone scan will not change the management and may not reveal any information that cannot be obtained from a detailed physical examination.

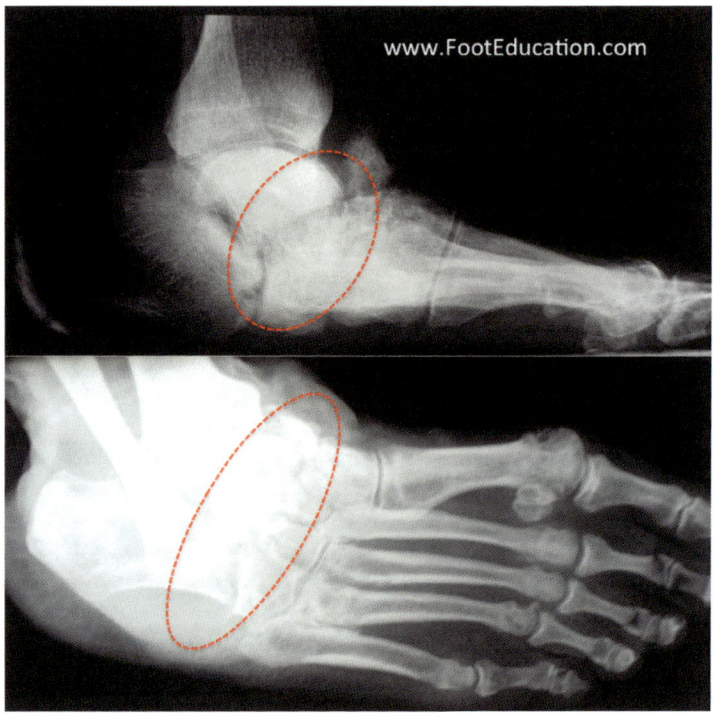

Figure 3: Lateral and Oblique x-rays of Charcot Arthropathy of the Transverse Tarsal Joint

In cases of suspected infection, aerobic and anaerobic cultures of the deep wound should be obtained to help direct antibiotic therapy. Osteomyelitis is present in approximately 70% of ulcers that extend down to bone.

Laboratory tests such as white blood cell counts, sedimentation rate, and C-reactive protein levels may be used to establish the diagnosis of osteomyelitis, though a bone biopsy is the most specific method.

CT scans can be helpful to look at a more detailed picture of the collapse, but is not often necessary unless surgery is planned.

EPIDEMIOLOGY

Diabetic foot disorders are a common subset of pathologies seen in patients with diabetes mellitus. The prevalence of diabetes in the US is approximately 10% of the adult population, and in turn, approximately 10% of those patients will develop a lower extremity ulcer during the course of their disease and about 1% will develop Charcot arthropathy.

The rate of lower extremity amputations is at least 50% higher in men versus women. Mexican (Hispanic) Americans, Native Americans, and African Americans each have at least a 1.5- to 2-fold greater risk for diabetes related amputations than age-matched diabetic Caucasians.

DIFFERENTIAL DIAGNOSIS

When a patient presents with a foot ulcer, it is essential to determine its cause. Thus, it is critical to evaluate foot ankle alignment and deformity, shoewear, assess for previous ulcerations, medical comorbidities, level of diabetic control and monitoring, and tobacco and intravenous drug use.

The presence of sensory neuropathy should be assessed. This can be done using a Semmes-Weinstein 5.07 monofilament to exert a consistent force (If the wire bows into a C shape when pressed against the skin for 1 second, 10g of force is applied). Sensation observed using the monofilament indicates protective sensation is maintained.

There are many potential causes for peripheral neuropathy besides diabetes. These can include: alcoholism, vitamin B1 and B12 deficiencies, and heavy metal poisoning. A focused history and appropriate laboratory studies can rule out other causes besides diabetes.

In the absence of diabetes, foot ulcers can be caused by atherosclerosis involving the lower extremities, vascular lesions, and even severe Raynaud's phenomenon (vasospastic attacks in digits). A squamous cell carcinoma may also be responsible.

Charcot arthropathy may have a similar presentation as gout, cellulitis, osteomyelitis, and septic arthritis. Diabetic neuropathy is the most common cause of Charcot arthropathy, but other less common causes include spina bifida, cerebral palsy, meningomyelocele, syringomyelia, leprosy, alcohol abuse, and advanced syphilis.

RED FLAGS

In all patients with diabetes, breaks in the skin are a red flag, as these can be a portal of entry for bacteria and subsequent infection. Any sign of increased pressure on focal areas of the foot (such as erythema or skin changes), is also considered a red flag and should be treated expeditiously.

TREATMENT OPTIONS AND OUTCOMES

The primary goal for treatment of diabetic ulcers is to get the wound to close and prevent future ulcerations. Off-loading of the affected area is an important first step in treatment of ulcers, commonly done using a total contact cast or removable diabetic walker boot (Figure 4). These allow healing by redistributing plantar pressure, decreasing shear stresses, and reducing swelling.

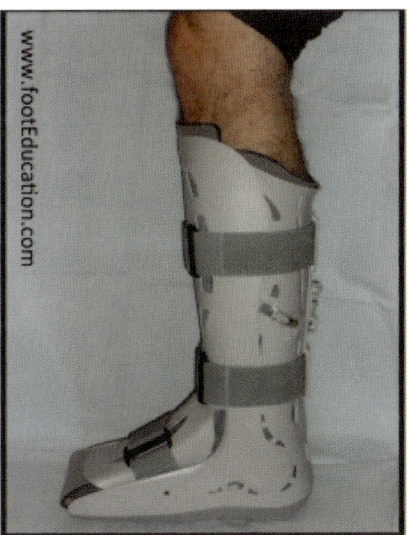

Figure 4: Removable diabetic walker boot used to reduce weight-bearing during ambulation

Total contact casting has been shown to significantly increase the healing rate of neuropathic plantar foot ulcers at 12 weeks compared to removable cast walkers and half-shoes so it is the preferred method of treatment. It can take anywhere from 6 weeks to a year for an ulcer to heal depending on the size, depth, and duration of the ulcer. A patient should not return to unmodified shoes until the ulcer has completely healed. Unfortunately, the highest risk factor for a second ulcer is having an initial diabetic foot ulcer even after successful healing. As a result, life long careful evaluation and protection is needed in these patients.

Treatment of the ulceration may involve surgical debridement of the callus or necrotic tissue with scalpels and curved scissors. Usually, this can be done in the clinic setting, although sometimes it may need to be done in the operating room if the infection involves the bone and there is some need to remove part of the infected bone. Keeping the wound moist without excess fluids can accelerate re-epithelialization of the wound. Various topical agents and dressings may expedite healing. Negative pressure wound therapy, hyperbaric oxygen therapy, ultrasonic therapy, and electric stimulation are all being tested for treatment of diabetic foot ulcers.

The vascular status of the affected extremity is critical in determining the healing potential of foot ulcers and the need for possible surgical intervention. More than 60% of diabetic foot ulcers have decreased arterial blood flow due to concurrent peripheral vascular disease. Formal vascular studies are often needed to determine status of the posterior tibial and dorsalis pedis arteries and the need for surgical or endovascular procedures to perfuse the foot.

Equinus contractures cause plantarflexion and thus increased forefoot pressures. Therefore a patient with an equinus contracture may benefit from a tendon release. A percutaneous Achilles tendon lengthening prior to total contact casting markedly decreases the rate of recurrence of plantar ulcers.

Diabetic foot ulcers if not treated (or if they do not respond to treatment) can lead to gangrene, abscesses, and osteomyelitis. Amputation of the lower extremity may be needed. An amputation is a marker for severe diabetic disease, as the 5-year mortality rate following an amputation in diabetic patients is approximately 66%.

Charcot arthropathy can be difficult to treat. The overall goal of Charcot arthropathy treatment is to maintain a braceable and plantigrade foot to allow ambulation and prevent ulcerations over bony prominences. The best approach is early detection and prevention. Early treatment consists of a period of non-weight-bearing or limited weight-bearing in either a total contact cast or a diabetic removable boot. Swelling and redness will usually resolve or improve with elevation and immobilization. Later in the process, bone consolidation will occur and the added stability can allow the patient to improve his mobility and weight-bearing. Rolling knee walkers can help keep the weight off the bad foot while allowing patients to be mobile. The treatment of Charcot arthropathy can take up to 6-12 months or more for the involved joints to stabilize. Even after consolidation of the Charcot process, gross bony deformity may be present that could put the patient at risk for developing an ulcer over those areas.

Some studies suggest that inhibitors of osteoclasts (as would be used to treat osteoporosis) may be helpful in treating Charcot arthropathy, by limiting osteolysis, though good clinical results have not yet been attained. Electrical bone growth stimulation to promote rapid healing of fractures has been suggested as a supplement to the treatment of acute Charcot arthropathy. Similar to bisphosphonate therapy, there is no conclusive data for its efficacy.

Surgery may be recommended as a treatment if a severe deformity has occurred that results in repeated ulcerations, non-plantigrade foot, or a foot or ankle that has become unstable and cannot be corrected through immobilization and off-loading. Surgery ranges from exostectomy (removal of prominent bone) to reconstruction of the foot including fusion of the unstable joints after the deformity has been corrected. The goal of surgery is a foot and ankle that is stable for weight-bearing, plantigrade, and can accommodate a diabetic shoe or brace. There are many risks for patients with Charcot arthropathy undergoing surgery such as infection, wound complications, non-union, delayed union, and hardware failure.

RISK FACTORS AND PREVENTION

Because diabetic foot disorders are caused by diabetes, all factors that increase the risk of the underlying condition increase the risk of resultant foot problems. Among patients with diabetes, cigarette smoking and poor glycemic control is associated with more diabetic neuropathy, peripheral artery disease, and in turn more foot disease. In addition, inappropriate footwear and poor toenail grooming increases the risk for ulcerations.

Previous ulcerations or amputations are associated with a higher risk of developing another ulcer.

A tight calf muscle (equinus contracture) causes the patient to place more weight on the forefoot and increases the risk of ulcers there.

MISCELLANY

There are reports of high complication rates associated with simple ankle fractures in the population of patients with diabetes, especially those with peripheral neuropathy. Many patients who present with Charcot arthropathy of the ankle initiated their disease process with an ankle fracture. Many experts recommend augmented internal fixation with prolonged non-weight-bearing to treat diabetic patients who have suffered an ankle fractures.

KEY TERMS

Diabetic foot ulcer, Charcot arthropathy, neurotraumatic theory, neurovascular theory, neuropathy, infection, amputation

SKILLS

Thorough physical exam of feet in diabetic population. Classify ulcers to treat accordingly. Distinguish infection from Charcot arthropathy. Provide basic patient education information to diabetic patients

CHAPTER 13.

CLUBFOOT

DESCRIPTION

Talipes equinovarus, commonly known as "clubfoot," is a congenital deformity of the foot (Figure 1). The condition is characterized by plantar flexion (equinus), inversion (varus), and an exaggerated arch (cavus) that may involve one or both feet. Taken together, these deformities cause the foot to resemble a club, hence the name. Clubfoot is often idiopathic and seen as an isolated birth defect, but it can also be caused by an underlying congenital disorder in approximately 20% of cases.

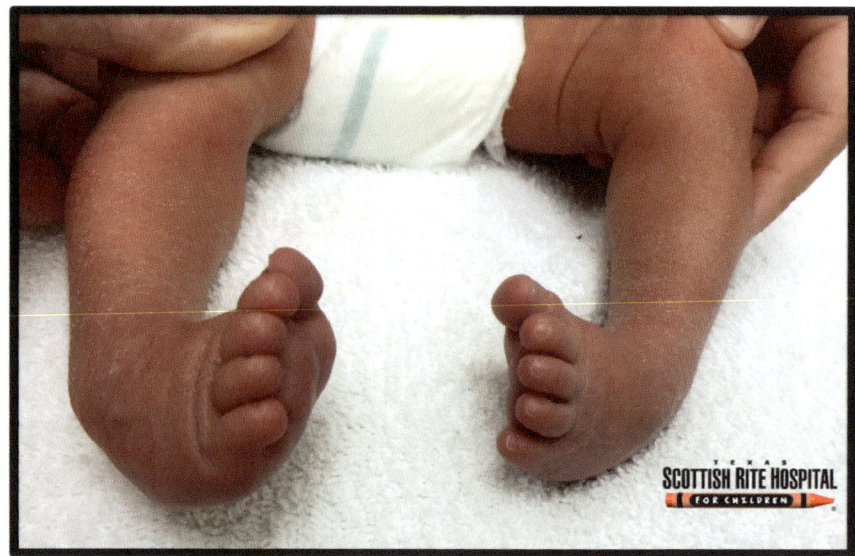

Figure 1: Bilateral clubfoot in a newborn with characteristic equinus and varus deformities. (Courtesy of Steve Richards MD, Texas Scottish Rite Hospital)

STRUCTURE AND FUNCTION

The foot can be divided into three regions: the hindfoot, the midfoot, and the forefoot.

The hindfoot consists of the talus and the calcaneus. These bones are joined at the subtalar joint to allow for inversion and eversion. The talus also articulates with the tibia and fibula at the ankle, to allow for dorsiflexion and plantarflexion.

The midfoot consists of the navicular, the cuboid, and the three cuneiform bones. The midfoot forms the arch of the foot and serves as a shock absorber.

The forefoot consists of the metatarsals and phalanges.

Clubfoot deformity primarily affects the hindfoot and midfoot. The pathological changes seen include an abnormally small calcaneus, talus, and navicular – and contracted ligaments between the hindfoot and midfoot. There is, accordingly, a plantarflexion deformity of the ankle (talocrural) joint, medial subluxation of the talonavicular and calcaneocuboid joints and inversion and adduction of the calcaneus, navicular, and cuboid.

The deformity can extend distally to the forefoot where there can be plantar flexion ("equinus") and adduction ("varus") of the metatarsals and proximally to the calf, with atrophy, fibrosis and shortening of the muscle-tendon units of the posteromedial leg muscles seen.

There are many theories about the etiology of clubfoot but the definitive cause is still unknown. In the past, experts believed that the deformity was caused by the foot being stuck in the wrong position in the womb; today it is known that clubfoot is associated with multiple genetic abnormalities that influence the muscle contractile complex and bone development. For example, Gurnett et al (PMID: 18950742) found that abnormalities of the PITX gene, responsible for early limb development, has been associated with familial clubfoot.

PATIENT PRESENTATION

Clubfoot is a congenital deformity that is immediately apparent at birth. Some parents might know as early as the second trimester if the clubfoot is diagnosed via fetal ultrasound.

The affected foot is characteristically adducted ("varus"), plantarflexed ("equinus"), and possesses an exaggerated arch ("cavus"). Depending on the severity, the foot may be rigid or flexible. Half of all cases will involve both feet. In unilateral clubfoot, the involved foot, calf, and leg will be smaller and shorter than the unaffected side. Even after correction of the deformity, the foot, calf, and leg may have some residual problems including atrophied calf muscles and a smaller foot that loads more on the outside.

Despite its dramatic deformities, clubfoot is not painful, per se. However, if children begin to walk prior to successful correction of the deformity, they will bear weight on the dorsolateral aspect of the foot. This abnormal gait can cause focal loading on a small area and can be painful.

OBJECTIVE EVIDENCE

Clubfoot is detectable via prenatal ultrasound in the second trimester. Early detection is important because it can prompt discussion with parents about treatment options and early screening for underlying neuromuscular diseases.

X-rays are not particularly useful in clubfoot evaluation because the neonatal bones are immature and poorly ossified. Radiographs are more useful for measuring progress in clubfoot treatment and long-term follow-up.

EPIDEMIOLOGY

Clubfoot occurs in 1 in 1000 births and affects males twice as frequently as females. Approximately 50% of all cases are bilateral and 25% have a positive family history of clubfoot. In the US, incidence ranges across ethnic groups from 0.4 in 1000 in the Chinese population to 7 in 1000 in the Polynesian population.

Most cases are idiopathic but about 20% are due to a genetic or chromosomal abnormality. The most common of these are disorders of the nervous system including myelomeningocele and arthrogryposis. These cases tend to be stiffer and more resistant to standard treatment than idiopathic cases.

DIFFERENTIAL DIAGNOSIS

Metatarsus adductus is a congenital foot deformity that is superficially similar to clubfoot. Metatarsus adductus is characterized by the forefoot (metatarsus) pointing inward (adductus) with normal positing and mobility of the hindfoot, forming a "C" shape. The incidence of metatarsus adductus is approximately the same as clubfoot. Metatarsus adductus is distinguished from clubfoot by an examination of the hindfoot, which has normal mobility in metatarsus adductus but cannot be appropriately dorsiflexed or everted in the case of clubfoot.

Other congenital foot deformities include talipes calcaneovalgus (dorsiflexed and abducted foot) and vertical talus (rigid foot deformity similar to talipes calcaneovalgus). These are structurally and visually distinct from clubfoot.

Certain conditions, including spina bifida, arthrogryposis, and amniotic band syndrome can cause clubfoot. The evaluator should therefore pay close attention to the spine and motor function of the extremities.

Positional clubfoot is similar to clubfoot in that the foot is in equinus and varus. It is caused by a restrictive uterine environment that forces the baby's feet into an abnormal position. However, it is different from classic clubfoot in that the foot and bony anatomy are completely normal.

RED FLAGS

Although clubfoot is most often an idiopathic birth defect, some cases are secondary to underlying neuromuscular conditions such as spina bifida. Thus, the presence of clubfoot should be deemed a red flag, prompting a close diagnostic evaluation to exclude these conditions.

TREATMENT OPTIONS AND OUTCOMES

Treatment options for clubfoot include serial casting, bracing, physical therapy, and surgery.

The standard of care for uncomplicated clubfoot deformities is the Ponseti Method, which involves repeated manipulation and casting (Figure 2) to guide the growth of the foot toward normal alignment. The child's foot is manually stretched toward the correct position and a cast is then applied to maintain the correction. This process is repeated weekly over the course of 4-6 weeks.

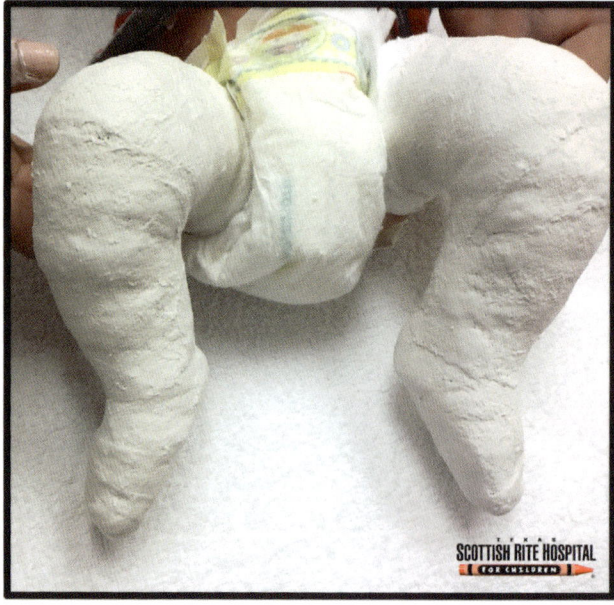

Figure 2: Clubfoot Cast (Courtesy of Steve Richards MD, Texas Scottish Rite Hospital)

Toward the end of the serial casting phase of treatment, most children will require a minor operation (percutaneous Achilles tendon tenotomy) to lengthen the Achilles tendon and release the foot from plantarflexion. Rarely, patients may also require a transfer of the tibialis anterior from its normal insertion on the first metatarsal to a new insertion on the third. This transfer will reduce supination of the foot with dorsiflexion. If the Ponseti Method of casting, bracing, and tenotomy is applied correctly, it will be successful in more than 95% of cases.

After casting, the child must wear a foot abduction brace (Figure 3) at night for a few years to maintain the correction. Without bracing, the deformity will likely recur because the muscles of the foot will pull it back into an abnormal position.

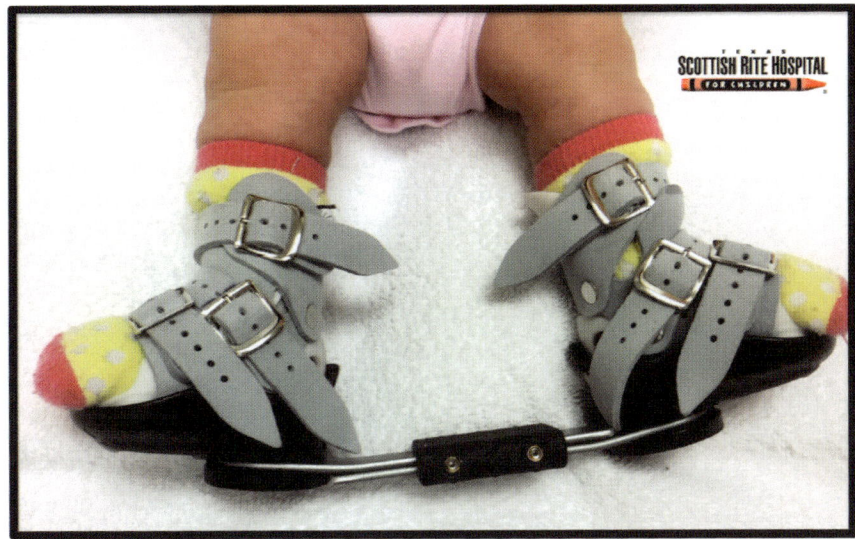

Figure 3: Abduction Bracing (Courtesy of Steve Richards MD, Texas Scottish Rite Hospital)

Recurrence (despite bracing) occurs in approximately 10% of patients, and most will respond to a repeated course of manipulation; a few will require additional surgery to prevent further relapse.

Although the Ponseti Method is highly effective in idiopathic clubfeet, some patients (especially those who present late or whose deformities are secondary to neuromuscular disease) will not respond to non-operative treatment and will require surgical intervention.

Surgery is normally performed at 9-12 months of age. The goal of surgery is to correct all the deformities in one operation. The surgical procedure varies from patient to patient but generally involves releasing all joint capsule contractures, lengthening any shortened muscle-tendon units, and realigning the bones of the foot.

Compared to the results of non-surgical methods, the long-term outcomes from surgery is associated with more pain, stiffness, deformity, and muscle weakness. However, it must be noted that surgery is reserved for tougher cases so this is not a true head-to-head comparison.

Even with optimal treatment, the corrected clubfoot will be functionally normal but structurally dissimilar from the unaffected foot. The affected foot is often smaller (requiring a different shoe size) and less mobile than the other foot. Additionally, the calf muscles in the affected leg may also be smaller. In some cases of clubfoot, the affected leg will stop developing before the other leg, leading to a significant difference in limb length. In these cases, it will be necessary to surgically lengthen the affected leg.

RISK FACTORS AND PREVENTION

Honien et al (PMID: 11032161) found that family history of clubfoot is a major risk factor for developing clubfoot (OR = 6.52). Smoking exposure in utero is also associated with increased risk of clubfoot (OR = 1.34). This risk is dramatically increased in babies that already have a past family history of clubfoot (OR = 20.30). As a result, mothers with a positive family history of clubfoot should be strongly urged not to smoke while pregnant to minimize the risk of their child having clubfoot.

Clubfoot can be identified in the second trimester using fetal ultrasound, which can help prepare parents for the treatment course and provide an opportunity for counseling about genetic testing for associated conditions.

MISCELLANY

Figure-skater Kristi Yamaguchi, soccer star Mia Hamm, and NFL quarterback Troy Aikman were all born with clubfeet but still attained great success as professional athletes.

Clubfoot is uniformly treated at a very early age in the US, but in low-income countries it is not uncommon to see older children with neglected clubfoot (a deformity that was never treated), residual clubfoot (a deformity that was incompletely treated and retains aspects of the deformity years later), and recurrent clubfoot (a deformity that was completely treated but reverted back due to insufficient bracing). These forms of clubfoot can severely decrease quality of life by subjecting patients to physical disability and alienation.

Horses walk on their toes; hence a deformity of plantar flexion that places the toes in lone contact with the ground is called "equinus."

KEY TERMS

Clubfoot, Talipes equinovarus, Ponseti Method

SKILLS

Recognize the gross manifestations of clubfoot and differentiate these from other congenital foot deformities. Explain treatment options for clubfoot, including the Ponseti Method of serial casting, bracing, and tenotomy. Describe the possible outcomes of clubfoot treatment, including restoration of normal form and function, residual deformity, and recurrent deformity.

PART III.

ACUTE FOOT AND ANKLE CONDITIONS

CHAPTER 14.

ACHILLES TENDON RUPTURE

DESCRIPTION

The most common acute injury to the Achilles tendon is a complete rupture. This injury typically occurs in men in their 30s and 40s. The inciting event often is an athletic activity that requires a sudden acceleration or changes in direction (ex. basketball, tennis, soccer). Ruptures typically occur 2 to 5 cm proximal to insertion into the calcaneus.

STRUCTURE AND FUNCTION

The Achilles tendon is the largest tendon in the body. The two main calf muscles, the soleus and gastrocnemius, coalesce to form the Achilles tendon, which then inserts into the posterior aspect of the calcaneus (Figure 1).

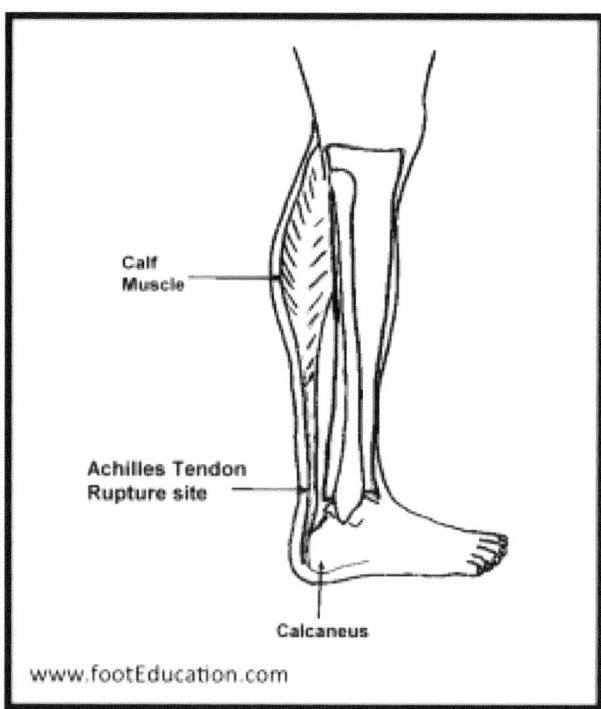

Figure 1: Achilles Anatomy

The Achilles functions to control the body as the center of gravity rotates over the foot. Without a functional Achilles, patients limp and have a markedly dysfunctional gait.

PATIENT PRESENTATION

Achilles tendon ruptures usually occur when an athlete loads the Achilles immediately prior to pushing off. This can occur when suddenly changing directions, starting to run, or preparing to jump (Figure 2). A sudden change in direction requires the calf muscle to contract while still lengthening (eccentric loading). This subjects the Achilles tendon to a large loading force, which may cause the tendon to fail. To be clear, the tendon tears because of the large internal forces generated by the eccentric contraction of the calf muscle and applied to the Achilles – and not because of an external force. In such a sense, it may be said that the patient tore the tendon himself. This explains why many patients feel as if they were "hit on the back of the leg" even though no one was around them when the injury occurred.

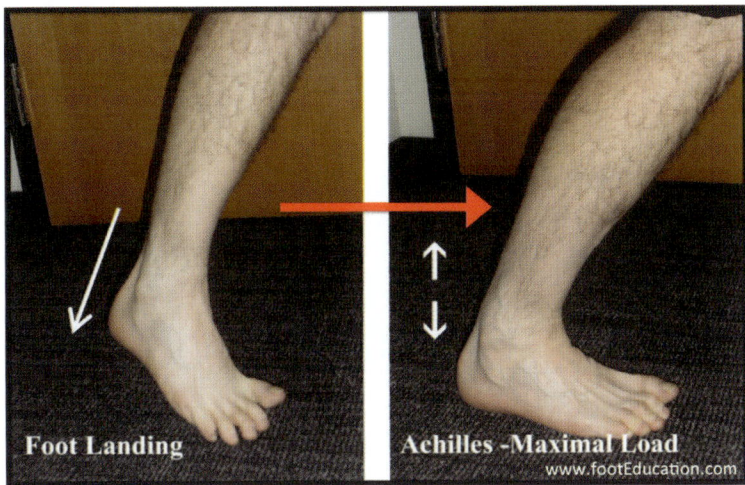

Figure 2: Achilles rupture mechanism of injury (Eccentric loading)

OBJECTIVE EVIDENCE

Achilles tendon tears are more common in middle-aged men who exercise intensely but intermittently (the so-called "weekend warrior"). With age the Achilles tends to lose flexibility and may develop areas of tendonosis (degenerative changes) that can serve to weaken the tendon.

A diagnosis of an Achilles rupture must be considered in any patient who reports an acute mechanism of injury (or acute change in symptoms) implicating the heel or soft tissues above it. In those patients, the examiner can exclude an Achilles tendon rupture) with the Thompson test. (Figure 3).

The Thompson test, as shown, takes advantage of the fact that squeezing the patient's calf muscles with the knee flexed should induce plantar flexion of the ankle if and only if the Achilles is intact. The patient lays prone on the examining table. The affected leg is flexed 90, perpendicular to the table (blue lines). The examiner firmly squeezes the gastrocnemius (black arrows). The examiner examines the ankle for plantar flexion

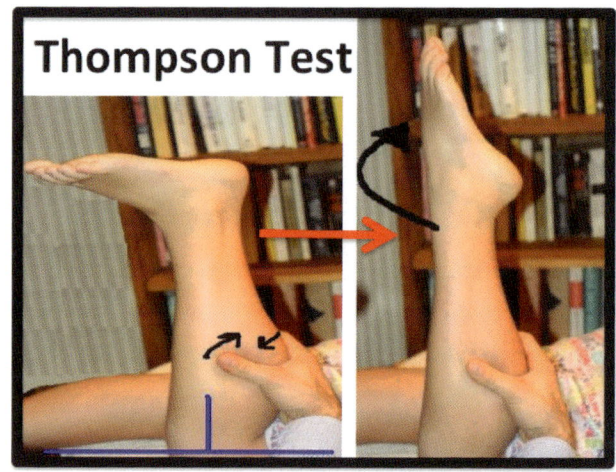

Figure 3: Thompson test: The Normal (negative) response, namely plantar flexion of the ankle produced by the examiner's pressure on the gastrocnemius, indicating that the tendon is NOT torn.

Two points are worth noting:

1. The nomenclature of the Thompson test can be confusing: a "positive" Thompson test is the absence of motion (whereas "positive" using means something was affirmatively observed). It is therefore helpful to describe the results as "positive for rupture" or "negative for rupture."
2. The Thompson test is necessary because testing active ankle plantar flexion can be misleading: an intact posterior tibialis and the flexors of the toe, which are both (weak) ankle flexors as well, might mask a torn Achilles. With these tendons intact, a patient with a ruptured Achilles may still be able to actively flex the ankle, especially without resistance.

A patient presenting with Achilles tendon rupture will often describe a sharp intense pain in the back of their heel at the time of the injury. Patients often initially report that they were "struck in the back of the heel" only to realize that this was not the case, as there was no one around them. After the injury, patients may have some swelling. If they can walk at all, it will be with a marked limp.

Note that Achilles tendonitis or a partial rupture of the calf muscle (gastrocnemius) as it inserts into the Achilles can also cause symptoms that suggest a tendon rupture. The Thompson test is helpful (indeed essential) here.

At times, an Achilles tendon rupture is obvious on physical examination: a substantial defect in the Achilles 2-5 cm proximal to where it normally inserts into the heel bone is appreciated, beyond the positive Thompson test.

IMAGING STUDIES

Plain x-rays will be negative in patients who have suffered an Achilles tendon rupture unless the Achilles injury involved an avulsion (traumatic displacement of a bony fragment from the calcaneus). Avulsions are rare, except in older patients with weaker bone.

Achilles rupture can be seen on ultrasound or MRI. However, these studies are usually not needed as a good history and well-performed physical exam should cinch the diagnosis. However, an MRI may be justified when the history or physical exam is ambiguous, or the quality of the tendon is in question (and whether it is amenable to repair) in the setting of chronic tendinopathy.

EPIDEMIOLOGY

Achilles tendon rupture is a common injury that occurs at an incidence of 2.66 per 1000 persons years or 18 per 100,000 population (PMID: 23386750). Middle-aged males are the largest group affected by this injury, and most injuries occur during athletic participation, most commonly basketball, soccer, or tennis.

RED FLAGS

Acute pain in the vicinity of the Achilles tendon or weakness of plantar flexion should be considered a "red flag" for an Achilles tendon rupture, prompting the examiner to perform the Thompson test.

TREATMENT OPTIONS AND OUTCOMES

Achilles tendon ruptures can be treated with either surgical repair or relative immobilization. If the ruptured tendon is ignored (or not correctly diagnosed) the tendon ends will retract, leading to failure of the calf muscle and a dysfunctional lower leg.

The medical literature suggests that ruptures treated with surgery are less likely to re-rupture, though there are complications (such as wound breakdown) that are unique to surgery. A published expected-value decision analysis on this issue reported that the optimal management strategy is highly dependent on patient preferences.

Non-Operative Treatment of Achilles Tendon Ruptures

Non-operative treatment consists of placing the foot in a downward position [equinus] initially, a position that encourages the torn ends to contact each other. Once there is some healing, the foot can be advanced to a more neutral position. Early weight-bearing and controlled active plantar flexion has been shown to improve non-operative treatment. However, care must be taken to avoid excessive dorsiflexion (extension), a position that encourages the torn ends to separate from each other.

It is important to monitor the status of the Achilles throughout non-operative treatment. This can be done by examination or via ultrasound. If there is evidence of gapping or non-healing, surgery may need to be considered.

The primary advantage of non-operative treatment is avoiding an incision in an area with a vascularity that puts the incision at higher risk for wound healing problems and infection. The main disadvantage of non-operative treatment is that the recovery appears to be somewhat slower and the re-rupture rate appears to be higher.

Operative Treatment of Achilles Tendon Ruptures

Operative treatment of Achilles tendon ruptures involves opening the skin and identifying the torn tendon. This is then sutured together to create a stable construct. By suturing the torn tendon ends together and assuring continuity even if the ankle is not in full plantar flexion, the patient can be mobilized more quickly.

RISK FACTORS AND PREVENTION

Factors that are associated with a higher risk for Achilles rupture include age between 30-50, male sex, playing recreational sports (most typically soccer, basketball, and tennis), prior steroid injections, and taking fluoroquinolone antibiotics.

KEY TERMS

Achilles tendon rupture; Thompson test

SKILLS

Bedside skills for the diagnosis of disorders of the Achilles include the ability to take a detailed but focused history and perform a thorough musculoskeletal examination. Specifically, students should be able to perform and interpret the Thompson test.

CHAPTER 15.

ANKLE SPRAIN

DESCRIPTION

Ankle sprains are among the most common musculoskeletal injuries. Patients typically describe an episode where they "roll their ankle" to one side (often inward, a so called "inversion" sprain (Figure 1) and thereby tear the ligaments on the outside (lateral) ankle. This is contrasted with a less common "eversion" sprain where the foot rolls to the outside and the medial (deltoid) ligament is torn. Patients with sprained ankles can have significant pain and swelling. There is usually a limp, but unlike an ankle fracture, a sprained ankle will usually tolerate some weight-bearing but, in severe cases, not for 7 to 10 days. Although the phrase "it's just a sprain" may suggest that this is always a minor injury, ankle sprains can in rare cases lead to significant impairment. Expeditious treatment – directed at limiting swelling and regaining motion – helps ensure the best possible recovery.

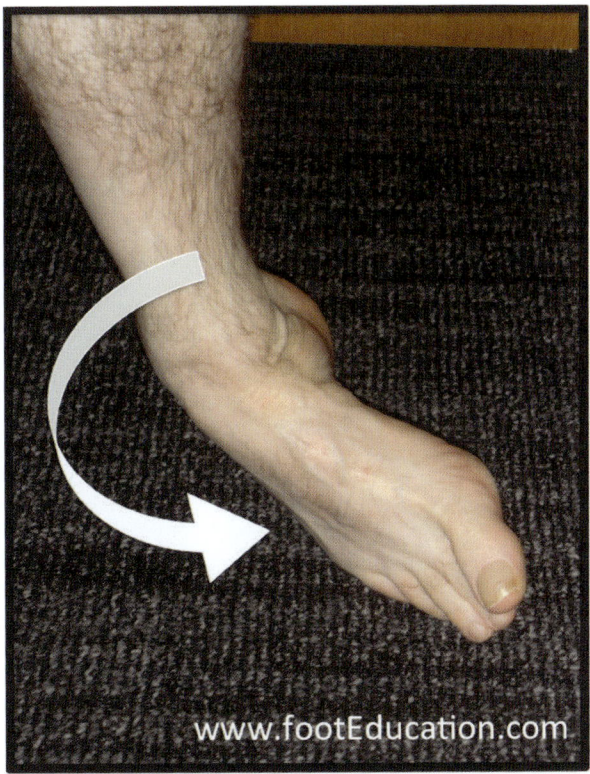

Figure 1: Ankle Inversion, the typical mechanism of injury of an ankle sprain

STRUCTURE AND FUNCTION

The ankle joint comprises the articulation of the tibia and fibula with the talus. However, the ligamentous constraints of the ankle also span the subtalar and talonavicular joints as well. The tibia and fibula are held together by the tibiofibular ligaments (anterior and posterior) and interosseous membrane, collectively known as the syndesmotic ligaments. These two bones form a mortise (inverted "U") into which the talus fits (Figure 2).

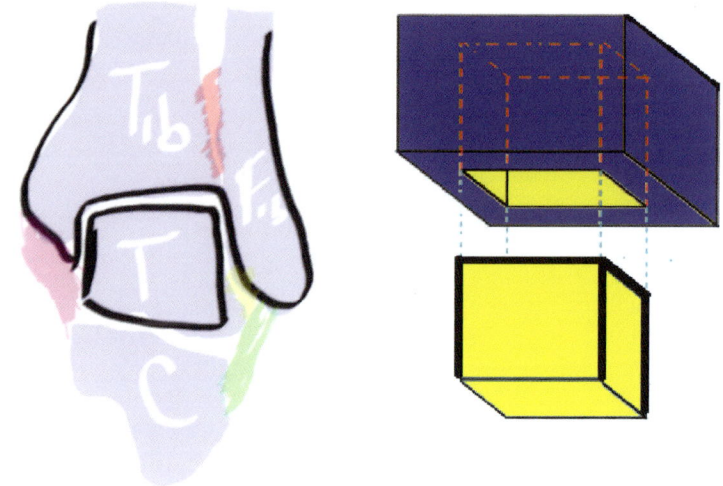

Figure 2: The Ankle Mortise. The talus (T) sits in an inverted U known as the mortise. The joint between the tibia (Tib) and fibula (Fib), the distal tibiofibular syndesosis. This relationship is vital to ankle function and is regulated by the anterior and posterior tibiofibular ligaments also referred to as the syndesmotic ligaments (shown in red). (Image courtesy of Joseph Bernstein MD)

The talus, in turn, acts as a "universal joint" that is connected to the calcaneus, forming the subtalar joint.

In addition to the syndesmotic ligaments, the ankle joint is stabilized, on the lateral side by the anterior and posterior talo-fibular ligaments and the calcaneofibular ligament, together referred to as the *lateral collateral ligaments* (Figure 3).

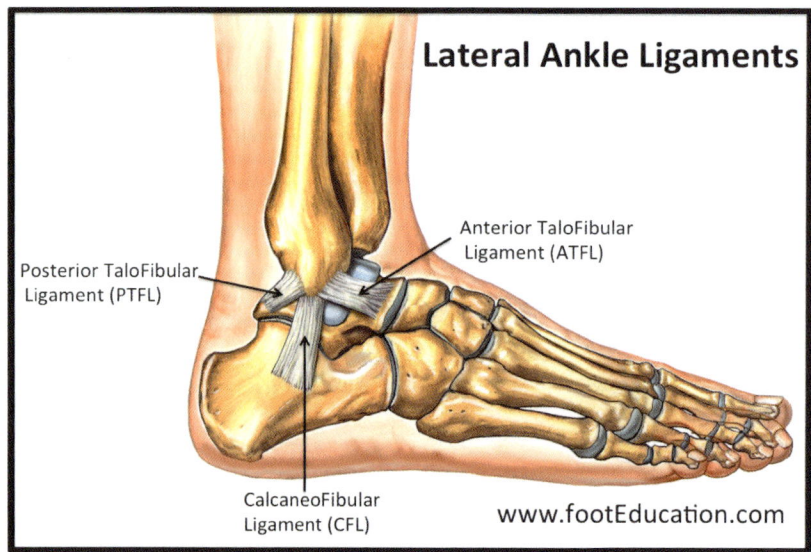

Figure 3: The Lateral Ligaments of the Ankle.

With its three parts, the deltoid ligament serves as the medial constraint of the ankle (Figure 4). The length and tension on these ligaments are vital to their role in the regulation of the *coupled motion* that occurs between the tibia, talus, calcaneus and navicular. The deeper branch of the ligament is securely fastened in the talus, while the more superficial, broader aspect runs into the calcaneus and navicular. Like the anterior talo-fibular ligament, the deltoid is rarely torn completely but rather becomes stretched (deformed) when stressed.

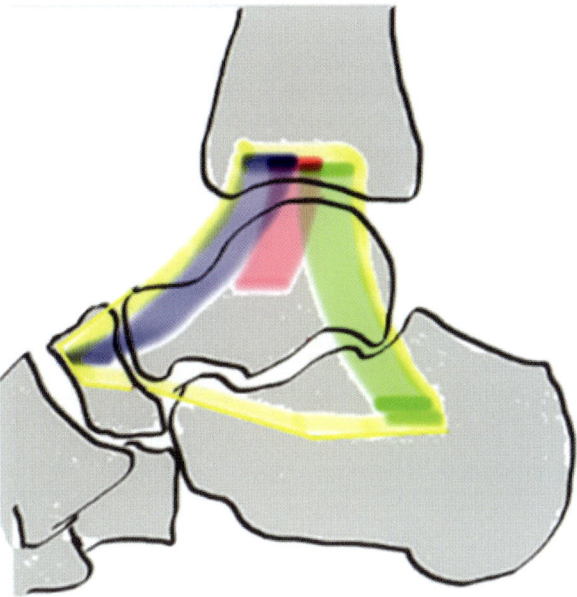

Figure 4: The Deltoid Ligament on the Medial Ankle The deltoid ligament is outlined in yellow (and shaped like a Delta). Within this ligament, there is a connection between the tibia and the navicular (blue), talus (red) and calcaneus (green). (Image courtesy of Joseph Bernstein MD)

The anterior talo-fibular ligament (ATFL) is the ankle ligament most often sprained. The ATFL courses from the fibula to the neck of the talus and stabilizes the ankle joint against anterior translation. Inversion of the ankle is resisted by a combination of the ATFL and calcaneo-fibular ligament. The ATFL itself is not a distinct ligament but, rather a thickening of the lateral joint capsule. When it is sprained, the associated interstitial tearing may result in lengthening. This stretching may lead to symptomatic ankle instability.

The calcaneo-fibular ligament (CFL) originates at the tip of the fibula and courses distal and posterior inserting into the calcaneus. Unlike the ATFL, the CFL is a distinct ligamentous structure.

The posterior talo-fibular ligament (PTFL) originates from posterior margin of the fibula and inserts into the posterior talus. The PTFL stabilizes the ankle joint and the subtalar joint. Injuries to the PTFL are rare, unless there is an ankle dislocation or marked subluxation.

The anterior inferior tibio-fibular ligament is the one injured in a so-called "high ankle sprain." This ligament is positioned on the anterolateral aspect of the ankle and helps stabilize the mortise (Figure 5). Injuries to this ligament occur when the foot is stuck on the ground and rotates externally. A high ankle sprain can heal with irritating scar formation (hypertrophy–a condition known as anterior-lateral ankle impingement.

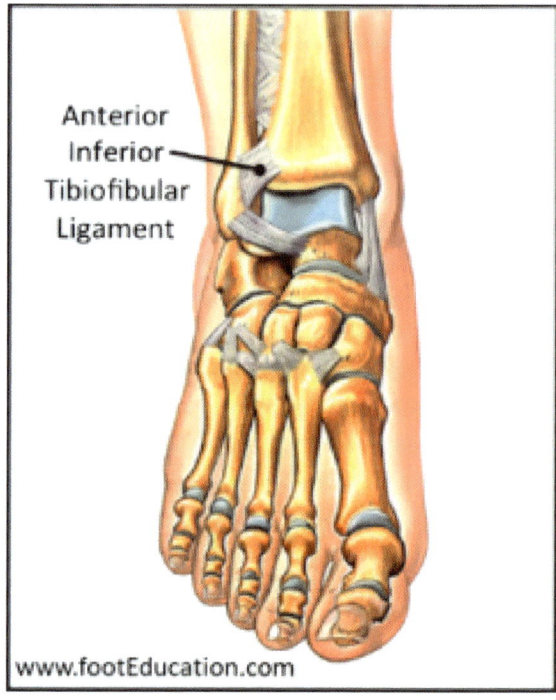

Figure 5: Anterior Inferior Tibiofibular Ligament

The interosseous membrane is composed of strong fibrous tissue that runs between and connects the tibia and fibula. The interosseous membrane along with the anterior or posterior syndesmotic ligaments can be torn in certain patterns of ankle fractures, in which the tibia and fibula spread apart, a so-called diastasis rendering the ankle unstable.

Collectively, the tibio-fibular ligament and the interosseous membrane are called the syndesmosis.

PATIENT PRESENTATION

Ankle Sprains

Patients with ankle sprains typically describe a twisting episode where they invert (or less often, evert) their ankle. Pain, swelling and difficulty ambulating are common.

A sprained ankle may often have associated redness due to the increased blood flow to this area (Figure 6). Without a history of an injury, this skin appearance may suggest cellulitis (infection of the skin). Physical examination of the acutely injured ankle will reveal swelling over the outer aspect of the ankle. There will be tenderness over the outer front (anterolateral) aspect of the ankle.

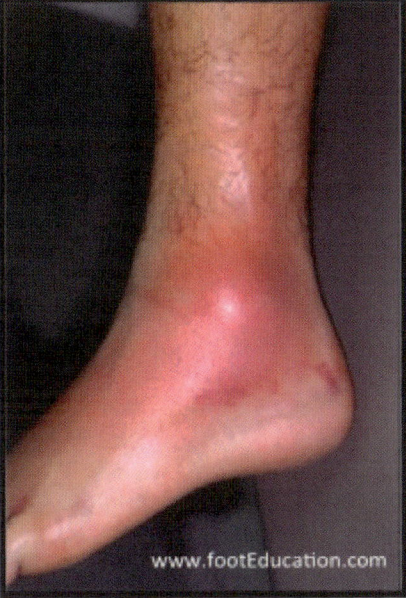

Figure 6: Ankle Swelling and Redness (erythema) Post-Ankle Sprain

It is important to palpate the base of the anterior process of the calcaneus, the 5th metatarsal, the navicular and the Lisfranc joint for tenderness, as the same mechanism that creates an ankle sprain can lead to other injuries there as well.

As swelling and pain decreases, during the recovery period it may be possible to assess for ankle instability. Laxity of the ATFL is assessed with an anterior drawer maneuver (Figure 7). Integrity of the calcaneofibular ligament is assessed by inverting the foot while palpating the lateral talar dome. Either or both of these tests can be obscured by guarding due to pain. The anterior draw test is performed on both the injured and uninjured side to obtain comparison. The examiner assesses the amount of translation of the foot relative to the shin and also the "quality of the end point" (i.e., if a firm stop —a rope snapping to attention— is encountered).

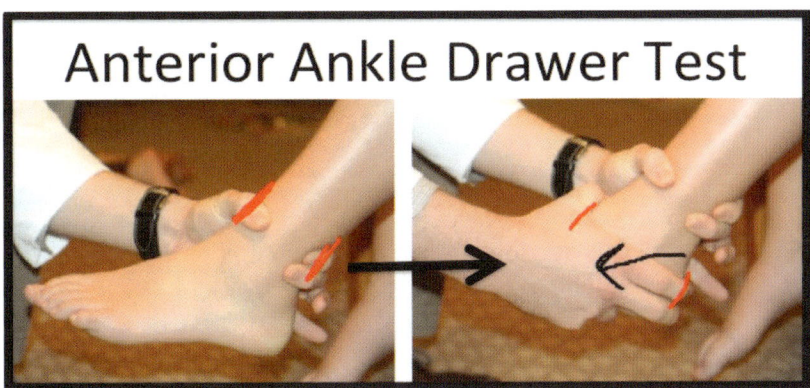

Figures 7: The Ankle Drawer Test

The anterior ankle drawer test is performed with the patient sitting on an exam table, with knees flexed and the foot dangling over the edge of the table. The examiner grasps and stabilizes the shin in one hand and applies anteromedial force to the heel with the other hand, using the deltoid ligament as a hinge.

High Ankle Sprains

So-called "high ankle sprains" are injuries to the syndesmosis, which lies between the tibia and fibula ("high") above the joint.

High ankle sprains are less common than lateral ankle sprains, but when they occur they are often more debilitating. They occur from a twisting injury to the ankle when the foot is planted on the ground. These injuries are produced by a sudden change of direction due to an externally applied force, as may be seen from a tackle in a football game. Pain located on the anterolateral aspect of the ankle is the main symptom. However, a high ankle sprain can also occur in combination with an inversion or eversion injury and therefore medial or lateral pain can be present as well.

The "squeeze test," namely compressing (squeezing) the tibia and fibula together approximately four inches above the ankle joint, can be used to detect a high ankle sprain. This test will tend to reproduce focal symptoms in patients who have had a high ankle sprain. The external rotation test, namely, holding the foot in dorsiflexion and then externally rotating it, will also reproduce focal symptoms when high ankle sprain is present.

OBJECTIVE EVIDENCE

X-rays should be obtained if there is bony tenderness on the posterior aspect of either malleoli or an inability to bear weight (Ottawa Ankle Rules). The x-rays should include the foot if there is tenderness on either the anterior process of the calcaneus, 5th metatarsal or the navicular. X-rays of the knee joint are needed if an isolated medial malleolus is detected on the initial film or if there is widening of the mortise (proximal fibular fracture can occur in combination with ankle injuries and must be ruled out).

X-rays must be examined to exclude not only fracture but diastasis, namely, an increased distance between the tibia and fibula implying damage to the syndesmosis.

Particular attention should be paid to ensure that the ankle joint mortise is symmetrical: the space between the talus and tibia medially should match the space laterally (Figure 8).

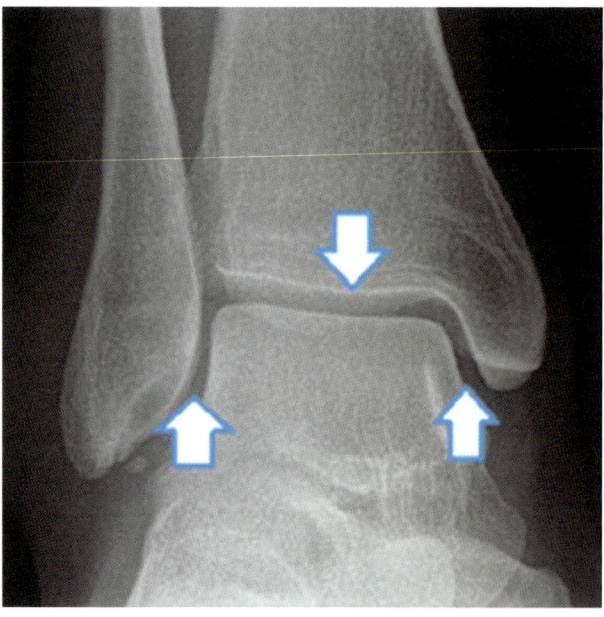

Figure 8: Talus Sits Squarely in the Mortise. The amount of space (arrows) should be uniform on all sides.

Stress x-rays – imaging the ankle while the heel is pushed towards one side while the leg is pushed in the opposite direction – may be used to assess instability in chronic cases. These films should be used only with great caution in the acute setting as the procedure may displace otherwise non-displaced injuries.

There is typically no role for MRI in acute ankle sprains. An MRI may be indicated in cases of chronic pain after a sprain. An MRI could detect a talar osteochondral injury or extra-articular sources of residual pain such as tendonitis or scarring of the restraining ligaments. Approximately 10% of severe ankle sprains may have associated injuries to the articular surface of the talus. An MRI may also be helpful in identifying an injury to the syndesmosis.

EPIDEMIOLOGY

According to Waterman et al (PMID: 20926721), emergency department data suggest an incidence rate of 2.15 ankle sprain per 1000 person/year in the United States, with a peak incidence rate more than triple that for teenagers between fifteen and nineteen years of age. The *overall* incidence rate by gender is about the same, though younger males and older females have higher rates than their female and male counterparts respectively. Nearly half of all ankle sprains seen were related to athletic activity.

DIFFERENTIAL DIAGNOSIS

The key element in the differential diagnosis of an acute ankle injury is discerning what was injured: which bones may have been broken and which ligaments may have been sprained. Note that combination injuries are not only possible but are common.

Bony tenderness on the anterior process of the calcaneus, base of the 5th metatarsal, or navicular suggests a fracture there.

Tenderness coursing up the lateral aspect of the leg may suggest a peroneal tendon injury.

The squeeze test and external rotation test may detect a high ankle sprain (anterior inferior tibia-fibular ligament injury).

Once the diagnosis of an ankle sprain is made, it can be further refined into a grade:

- *Grade 1 sprain:* the anterior talofibular ligament is injured but not elongated (and thus not prone to cause instability);
- *Grade 2 sprain:* the anterior talofibular ligament is partially torn resulting in stretching that may destabilize the joint; and
- *Grade 3 sprain:* a complete tear of the anterior talofibular ligament. Note that instability may be masked by swelling or guarding.

RED FLAGS

An inability to bear weight or tenderness in the bone (including the medial and lateral malleoli as well as the 5th metatarsal and navicular) signify a need for radiographs (as per the Ottawa Ankle Rules).

Blood on the skin suggests an open fracture.

TREATMENT OPTIONS AND OUTCOMES

The initial treatment of an ankle sprain is known by the mnemonic RICE. RICE is used to limit swelling, as too much swelling can significantly increase the patient's pain and ultimate recovery time.

- **R**est: minimize mobilization and activity in the initial recovery period.
- **I**ce: Apply ice, but not continuously. A regimen of 10 minutes on and 10 minutes off will minimize the risk of thermal injury to the skin.

- **Compression:** This should be tight enough to decrease swelling but loose enough to allow the foot to be perfused.
- **Elevation:** To be maximally effective, the foot should be held higher than the thigh, to allow gravity to help drain the edema. Propping the foot in a stool or pillow is not apt to help drain fluid, but may help enforce rest and inactivity.

Non-Steroidal Anti-Inflammatory Drugs (NSAIDs) such as ibuprofen can be very helpful to decrease pain by decreasing the inflammatory response to the injury. However, there is some evidence that suggest that anti-inflammatories may have an adverse effect on ligament healing.

Once the symptoms associated with the initial ankle sprain have started to improve, patients will benefit from *physical therapy exercises* designed to improve their range of motion, strength and proprioception.

Proprioception is the ability of the brain to sense the position of a joint (ex. ankle) and control its movement relative to the rest of the body. Note that nerves within the ligament mediate proprioception and therefore this sense can be out of kilter following a ligament injury. As the acuity of the injury resolves, patients with seemingly normal ankles on examination (no swelling, no tenderness, no laxity) may still feel unstable if proprioception has not returned to normal. This is referred to as "functional instability."

"Figure of Eight" exercises are particularly helpful for regaining range of motion and proprioception. Patients should be instructed to imagine that the tip of their big toe is a pen and to then "draw" a figure of eight with the toe slowly, repeating the motion for 30-60 seconds. In the alternatives, patients can "sign" their names in script. It is important that the motion follow a deliberate pattern – and not random waving of the foot – as deliberate motion helps improve proprioception as well.

Proprioception can also be improved by having the patient stand on one foot with eyes closed. Once this is mastered, standing on one foot on a soft surface (such as a pillow or bed) with eyes closed and head moving side to side can further improve proprioception.

Rehabilitation after an ankle sprain can often be completed with a home program, though trained physical therapists may be beneficial in providing initial instruction defining the program.

Surgery is rarely indicated for the treatment of acute ankle sprains. However, patients who have recurrent ankle sprains may be candidates for an ankle ligament stabilization procedure to treat their anatomic instability and restore functional stability.

Most people with sprained ankles fully recover. Even if the ligaments are permanently deformed, the muscles crossing the ankle joint can provide sufficient dynamic stability. However, because ankle sprains are such a common injuries, even a low rate of complications (coupled with a high incidence) may produce a significant number of people with poor outcomes. Ankle injuries associated with chronic anatomic instability may lead to the development of traumatic arthritis.

RISK FACTORS AND PREVENTION

Risk factors for ankle sprains include a high arched foot (cavus foot), ligamentous laxity leading to increased inversion, participating in high risk activities (ex. basketball, soccer, volleyball), and a history of previous ankle sprains.

Rovere et al (PMID: 3132864) studied the effectiveness of taping, wearing a laced stabilizer and high-top or low-top shoes among collegiate football for 6 seasons. They reported that the combination associated with the fewest injuries overall was low-top shoes and laced ankle stabilizers.

MISCELLANY

Ankle sprains from playing basketball represent nearly 20% of all ankle sprains in the US. Football and soccer are the next most implicated sports causing ankle sprains during athletics.

KEY TERMS

Ankle sprain, syndesmosis, mortise, talo-fibular ligament, calcaneo-fibular ligament, deltoid ligament, proprioception

SKILLS

Recognize an ankle sprain and differentiate between it and other ankle and hindfoot injuries. Apply the Ottawa ankle rules to recognize need for x-rays.

CHAPTER 16.

ANKLE FRACTURES (TIBIA AND FIBULA)

DESCRIPTION

Ankle fractures are breaks of the distal tibia or fibula (near or in the so-called malleolus) affecting the tibiotalar (ankle) joint. Occasionally, they involve the shaft of the fibula as well. Ankle fractures range from simple injuries of a single bone to complex ones involving multiple bones and ligaments. Twisting with the foot planted on the ground and the body rotating around it is the most common mechanism of injury. Compression loading (ex. from a fall) is more apt to produce a fracture of the weight-bearing surface of the distal tibia (the plafond). These are designated as "pilon fractures," and are considered distinctly different injuries. Ankle fractures can be broadly divided into stable or unstable injuries. Stable fractures typically heal with immobilization and protected weight-bearing whereas operative management is usually required for displaced or unstable fractures. Ankle fractures directly or indirectly involve the ankle joint. Some residual ankle arthrosis is therefore not uncommon, even if the bone heals perfectly.

STRUCTURE AND FUNCTION: ANKLE ANATOMY

The ankle joint is made up of the tibia, fibula, and talus (Figure 1). The tibia forms the superior and medial aspects of the joint, and the fibula its lateral aspect. The talus is a cube-shaped bone that sits above the calcaneus and below the tibial plafond. The distal ends of the fibula and tibia that overlap the talus are known as the malleoli ("little hammers"). The lateral malleolus is the distal end of the fibula, whereas the medial and posterior malleoli are part of the tibia. A fracture affecting both the medial and lateral malleoli is called a bimalleolar fracture, and one involving the medial, lateral, and posterior malleoli, the posterior aspect of the distal tibia, is called a trimalleolar fracture.

The ankle joint also contains three important ligament complexes:

1. The deltoid ligament medially, connecting the tibia to the talus and calcaneus medially.
2. The anterior and posterior talo-fibular, and calcaneo-fibular ligaments (collectively, the lateral collateral ligaments); and
3. The anterior and posterior distal tibiofibular ligaments or syndesmosis, which connects the distal tibia and fibula above the tibio-talar joint line.

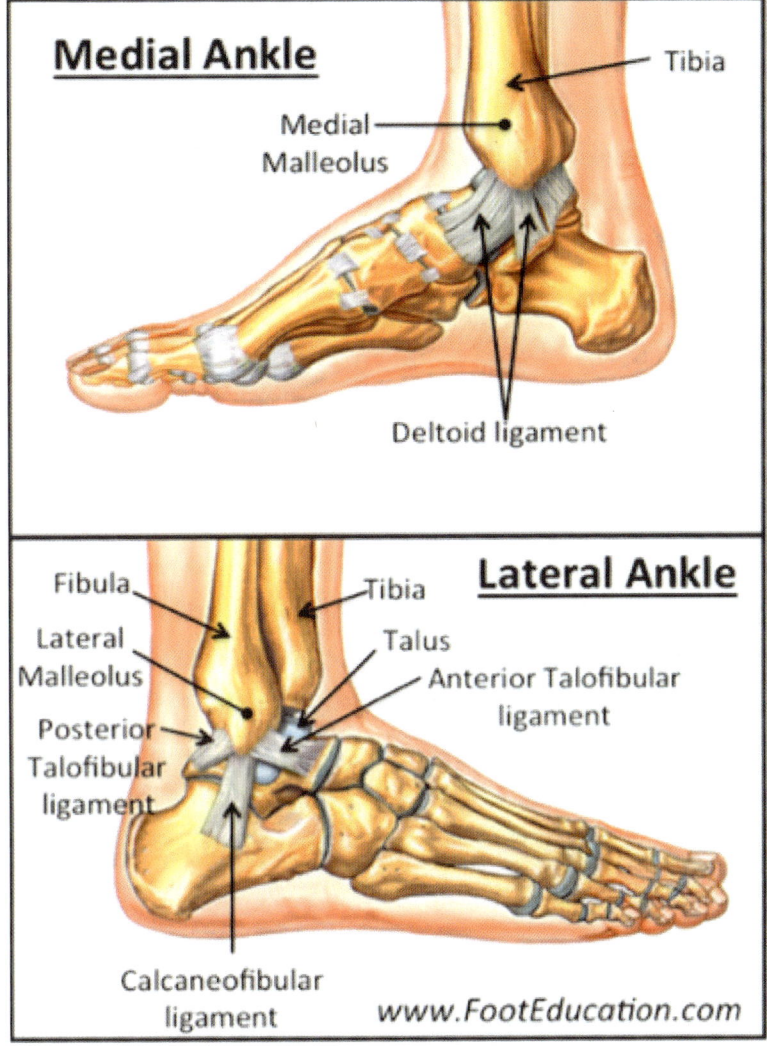

Figure 1: Bone and Ligament Anatomy of the Ankle Joint.

The tibial plafond, lateral malleolus, and medial malleolus form a mortise, a socket in which the talus sits (Figure 2). Although the ligaments are needed to give the ankle its full stability, the bony congruity of the mortise and the talus is a necessary component as well forming the most congruent joint in the lower extremity.

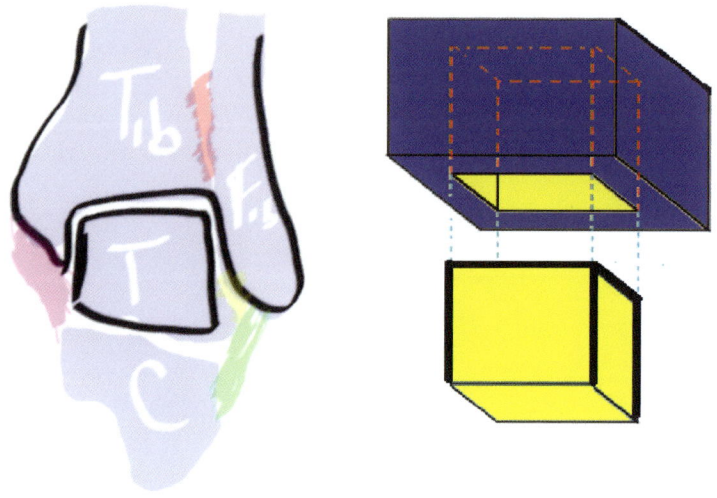

Figure 2: The Ankle forms a Mortise and Tenon (carpentry version shown at right). The mortise (the socket) comprises the lateral malleolus, the tibial plafond, and the medial malleolus. The tenon (or tongue) is the talus. As seen, the talus is wedged into a space just big enough to hold it. (Image courtesy of Joseph Bernstein MD)

When the mortise is disrupted by a fracture, the talus is free to move more than it should. This abnormal motion leads to focal pressure points which can be damaging. Recall that pressure is defined by the force (load) divided by area. Thus, a smaller area of contact for a given load leads to higher pressure. This pressure produces new bone. This is in accordance with Wolff's Law, which states that bone grows in response to load. This new bone in turn makes the tissue below the cartilage more rigid (technically speaking less compliant). The loss of compliance makes the entire system more prone to damage. The surface may crack and not bend in response to a new load.

Ankle Fracture Classifications

There are many methods of classifying ankle fractures: some are too simple (and therefore not very informative), and others provide more detailed information (yet become unwieldy and unreliable). It may be best, therefore to describe ankle fractures by the bones involved (i.e., isolated medial/lateral malleolar, bimalleolar, trimalleolar, etc.) and the presence of absence of soft tissue injury. Regarding the soft tissues, the single most important feature to note is whether the fracture is "open," that is, that the skin is broken.

Another important consideration is the stability of the ankle joint (Figure 3). Ankle fractures are classified as stable if the fracture is non-displaced or minimally displaced and the medial structures (deltoid ligament and medial malleolus) are intact. This type of injury allows the talus to remain anatomically positioned within the mortise, preventing displacement of the joint.

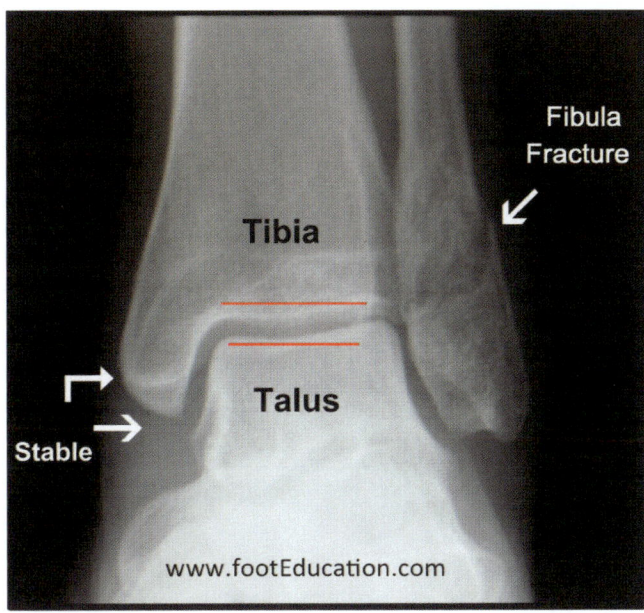

Figure 3: Plain X-Ray of a Stable Ankle Fracture. Note the mortise is intact: the space surrounding the talus is normal.

Ankle fractures are unstable if the injury allows the talus to be move within the mortise (Figure 4).

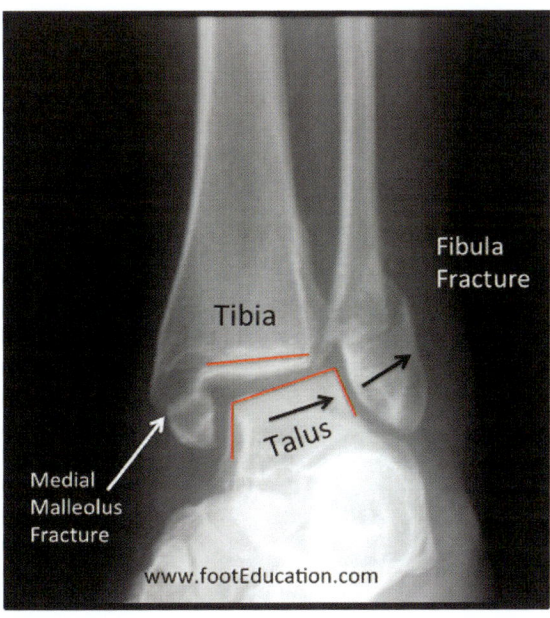

Figure 4: Plain X-Ray of an Unstable Ankle Fracture. Note how the talus is displaced laterally along with the fibular fragment and no longer sits snugly within the distorted mortise.

The fracture pattern often provides useful clues not only regarding the mechanism of injury but whether there are associated lesions (that may not be apparent on the x-ray). For example, a transverse fracture is produced by traction from ligaments pulling on the bone (Figure 5). Yet for this traction force to be produced, the foot must move medially, perhaps creating an impact on the medial side. Similarly, a fracture caused by a rotational ankle injury will often produce a spiral-type fracture of the distal fibula (Figure 6). This fracture pattern is associated with tearing of the anterior inferior tibiofibular ligament and possibly partial or complete injury to the deltoid ligament on the medial aspect of the ankle.

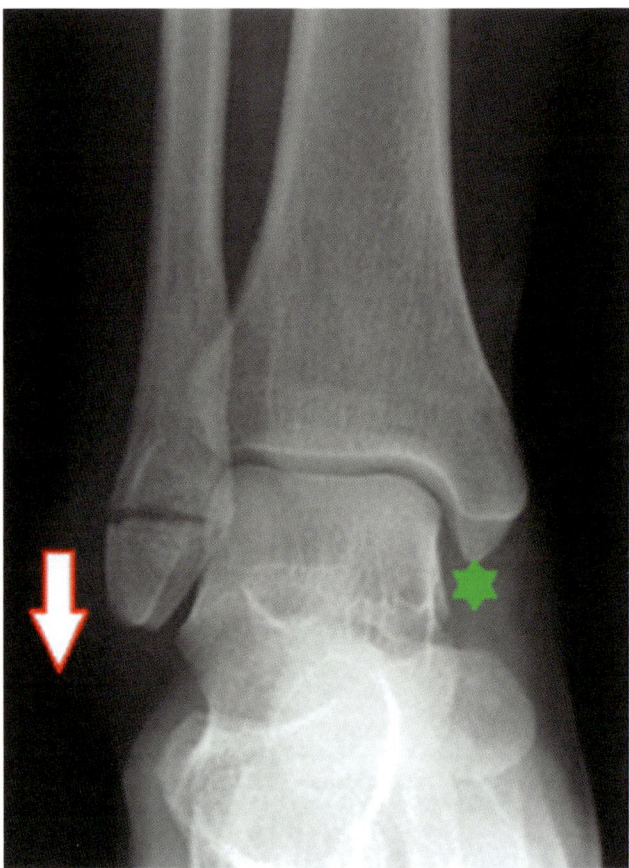

Figure 5: A Transverse Fracture of the Distal Fibula. This fracture is produced by a traction force, depicted by the arrow. The motion of the foot needed to produce this force may cause the talus to hit the tibia medially, producing a bone bruise if the force is mild (as shown by the star) or even a fracture on this side as well (not shown).

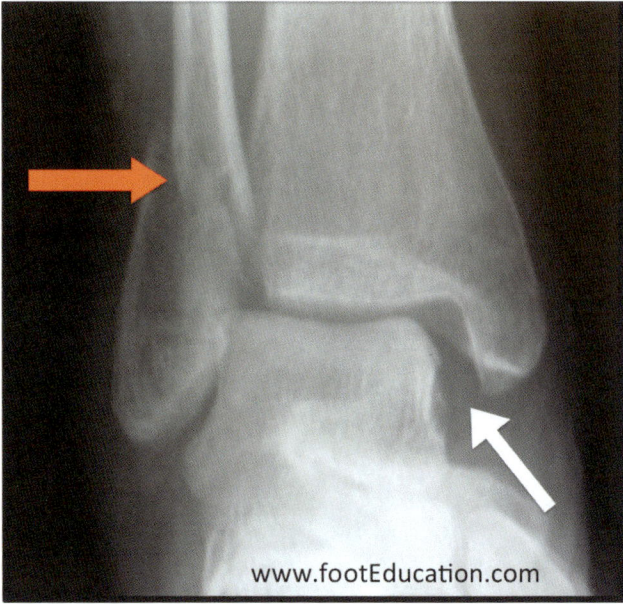

Figure 6: Oblique Fracture of the Fibula (red arrow) Produced by Twisting.

This force also applies traction to the deltoid ligament on the medial side. Although the deltoid ligament cannot be "seen" on the x-ray, the injury is easily inferred, given the widening of the mortise nearby (white arrow).

PATIENT PRESENTATION

Patients with ankle fractures usually present with pain, swelling, and bruising. Patients typically describe an acute twisting injury in which the foot is planted on the ground and the body rotates around it.

The direction of rotation, the orientation of the foot while planted and the amount of energy that produces the fracture will determine which bones and ligaments may be injured. While this is useful information to obtain, it is often the case that the patient cannot recall or describe exactly what happened. Nonetheless, it is important to obtain a history of the general mechanism of injury, to help guide further investigation. For example, ankle pain after a fall from a height or a motor vehicle crash is likely to be from force transmitted from the heel up the leg, and therefore injury to the calcaneus, talus, tibial plafond, and more proximal bones (including even the spine) must be considered.

OBJECTIVE EVIDENCE

Patients with suspected ankle fractures should have x-rays performed: an anterior-posterior (AP), lateral, and mortise view. A mortise view is an AP view with the foot slightly internally rotated (about 15 degrees) which produces a clearer view of the mortise (Figure 7). These views should be evaluated for the integrity of the bones as well as proper alignment between joint surfaces.

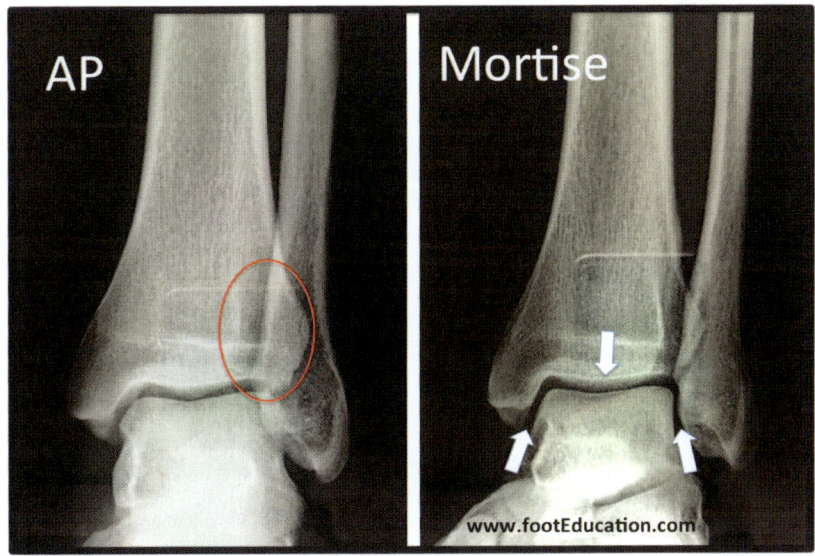

Figure 7: Mortise View of the Ankle (right). Internal rotation of the foot will give a clearer view of the mortise. Without such rotation (AP view left), the fibula, which is slightly posterior, will overlap with the tibia (red circle) making it difficult to assess the symmetry of the joint space (white arrows).

Not all patients with ankle injuries should be "suspected" of having an ankle fracture. Indeed, according to one study (PMID: 15496699) of acute ankle injuries in the Emergency Department, sprains outnumber fractures by an 8:1 ratio. To help guide the decision whether ankle x-rays are needed, the Ottawa Ankle Rules have been developed. According to these rules, ankle radiographs are not necessary if posterior malleolar (bony) tenderness is absent, and the patient can bear weight (take more than four steps).

In some patients, an unstable ankle fracture is only diagnosed after the ankle is "stressed" under x-ray revealing the lateral displacement of the talus and therefore disruption of the deltoid ligament or syndesmosis.

EPIDEMIOLOGY

According to Lin et al (PMID: 21655420), ankle fractures occur in the USA with an incidence of approximately 187 fractures per 100,000 people per year. Fracture incidence by age is bimodal, with men typically having higher rates as young adults and women having higher rates as elderly adults. The highest incidence is found in elderly white women.

The most common type of ankle fracture is an isolated fibular fracture, representing about half of all ankle fractures. One-fourth of ankle fractures are bimalleolar, while trimalleolar fractures and isolated medial malleolar fractures are less common. Only 2% of ankle fractures are open.

DIFFERENTIAL DIAGNOSIS

When a patient presents with an acute ankle injury, it is necessary to discern which structures have been damaged.

Injuries that cause ankle fractures may also cause damage outside of the ankle region per se. For example, a twisting injury to the foot and ankle may send force through the syndesmosis and interosseous membrane, up the leg. This can lead to a fracture of the proximal fibula near the knee — a so-called Maisonneuve fracture (Figure 8). This injury is produced by a strong external rotation force, one that would assuredly damage the lateral side of the ankle as well. Yet no fibular injury is seen *near the ankle.* In this case, the lateral injury was to the proximal fibula. This injury is important to detect given the proximity of the common peroneal nerve to the fibular fracture line. While this type of high fibula fracture requires no treatment to heal adequately, the associated syndesmotic disruption and deltoid ligament disruptions usually require surgery to ensure precise reduction and stabilization of the syndesmosis.

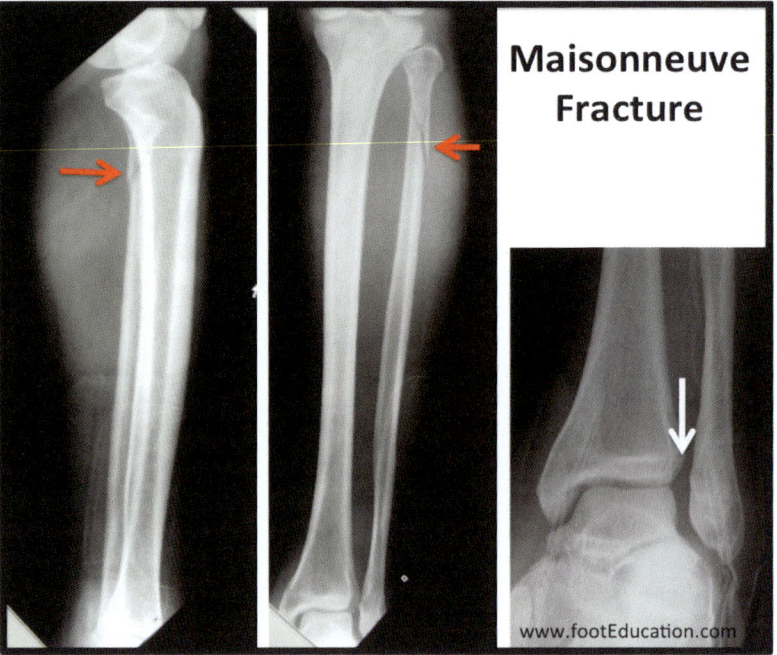

Figure 8: Maisonneuve Fracture. Note the proximal fibula fracture (red arrow) and the widened syndesmosis (white arrow).

Foot injuries involving the tarsometatarsal (Lisfranc) joint, the navicular bone or posterior tibial tendon, or the fifth metatarsal can easily be missed if attention is paid to only the ankle joint itself.

RED FLAGS

Blood on the skin is suggestive of an open fracture. Any break in the skin associated with an ankle fracture should be considered an open fracture until proven otherwise. Open fractures require administration of antibiotics and tetanus prophylaxis as indicated. Basic wound management (cleaning the wound with saline and applying a dressing and splint) should not await the arrival of a specialist.

If a patient presents with severe ankle pain following an acute injury but x-rays are normal, an injury to the foot and not the ankle, such as a Lisfranc joint disruption or navicular fracture, may be present.

Diabetic patients, especially if their diabetes is uncontrolled (HgA1C >7%), have a much higher risk of complications and need close attention.

If a patient's growth plates are open, a non-displaced physeal fracture should be suspected if there is bony tenderness, despite "normal" x-rays.

The presence of a pilon fracture should prompt a careful physical examination to exclude addition injuries more proximally such as a lumbar compression fracture.

TREATMENT OPTIONS AND OUTCOMES

All dislocations should be reduced (that is, realigned).

Open wounds should be cleaned and dressed; and prophylactic antibiotics (and a tetanus shot, if indicated) should be given.

The ankle should then be immobilized with a splint and elevated to minimize swelling.

If the fracture is stable and not displaced, a course of immobilization and protected weight-bearing for about 6 weeks may suffice. Following adequate bone healing, physical therapy can help the patient regain strength, range of motion, and proprioceptive function.

Operative fixation will be necessary if there is notable displacement of the bone fragments or the injury has caused a disruption of the ankle mortise. Surgery generally consists of making incisions at the affected malleoli, re-positioning the bony fragments to their appropriate positions, and holding them in place with screws and plates (Figure 9). The primary goal of surgery is to ensure that the talus is anatomically reduced and stable within the ankle mortise. The hardware can be left in the joint permanently unless it causes irritation, in which case it can be removed once the fracture has healed.

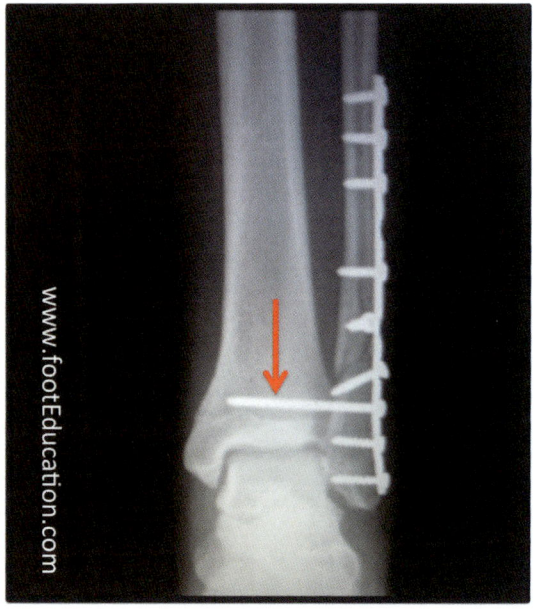

Figure 9: Ankle Fracture Fixation with a Plate and Screws.

The longer screw (arrow) into the tibia is used to stabilize the syndesmosis and thereby reduce the ankle mortise by holding the tibia and fibula in the correct position to allow the ligaments that normally stabilize the ankle joint to heal.

Outcomes for stable fractures treated non-operatively are generally excellent. Ankle fractures treated with operative fixation heal uneventfully in approximately 85% of the cases. Not surprisingly, outcomes improve with more accurate reduction. Factors that negatively affect outcomes include involvement of the posterior malleolus, impaction of the talus, severe talar dislocation, and the presence of diabetes. Recovery time will depend on the severity of the initial injury but it often takes a year or more before patients reach their point of maximal improvement. Even then, mild to moderate symptoms may persist for years despite complete radiographic healing.

Complications of ankle fractures include malunion, non-union, stiffness, and wound breakdown.

Even with optimal treatment, some ankle fractures may result in post-traumatic ankle arthrosis as damage to the articular surface at the time of injury can lead to chondrocyte death. The likelihood of post-traumatic ankle arthritis increases with the severity of the initial ankle fracture.

Sub-optimal reduction of the joint and resultant abnormal biomechanics will also promote the development of ankle arthrosis.

Another possible, albeit rare, complication of ankle fractures is complex regional pain syndrome (CRPS; previously known as reflex sympathetic dystrophy or RSD). This uncommon but debilitating condition is characterized by burning or throbbing pain, sensitivity to cold or touch, weakness, stiffness, and changes in skin color, temperature, or texture.

RISK FACTORS AND PREVENTION

Valtola et al and Honkanen et al (PMID: 11792591, 9692074) found that risk factors for the occurrence of ankle fracture in perimenopausal woman are cigarette smoking and a high body mass index. According to Seeley et al (PMID: 8864910), although low bone density is a risk factor for other fractures, it has not yet been shown to be a major risk factor for ankle fractures in this patient population.

MISCELLANY

Just as a piece of masking tape yanked briskly from a wall may take with it a sliver of paint as well, a sprained ligament may yank with it a small sliver of bone — a so-called avulsion fracture. The finding is important only that it informs the viewer that a sprain has occurred. The bony injury is itself insignificant, but patients will still often identify this injury as a "fractured ankle."

KEY TERMS

Ankle fracture, Maissoneuve fracture, Lateral malleolus, Medial malleolus, Posterior malleolus, Ottawa Ankle Rules, Mortise, Syndesmosis, Tibial plafond, Bimalleolar fracture, Trimalleolar fracture, Pilon fracture.

SKILLS

Perform an exam to determine the extent of injury and structures involved. Apply the Ottawa Ankle Rules to decide which patients require radiographic evaluation. Describe radiographic findings and use radiographs to identify fractures, infer ligamentous injuries, and recognize instability and displacement. Differentiate between stable and unstable ankle fractures. Provide first-line treatment to open fractures (wound management) and dislocations (gross reduction and splinting).

CHAPTER 17.

MIDFOOT TRAUMA: LISFRANC INJURIES

DESCRIPTION

An injury to the tarsometatarsal joint is known by the eponym "Lisfranc injury." These types of injuries include sprains of the midfoot ligaments, fractures, or a combination of the two. Midfoot trauma including Lisfranc injuries are relatively rare, but when they occur they can be severe. Symptoms include marked pain, swelling, and inability to bear weight. Some Lisfranc injuries are subtle and can go undetected at first. Because these untreated injuries can be disabling, it is essential to diagnose them as they occur.

STRUCTURE AND FUNCTION

The midfoot (navicular, cuneiforms, and cuboid tarsal bones) meets the metatarsals at the tarsometatarsal joint, also known as the Lisfranc joint complex (Figure 1). This joint is stabilized by strong ligaments, particularly the plantar ligaments which support the arch and markedly limit motion through the joints of the midfoot. Bony congruence is also critically important to stability of the tarsometatarsal joint – namely, the articulation of the cuneiforms and bases of the metatarsals. The keystone of this arch is the base of the second metatarsal, which is tightly recessed between the medial and lateral cuneiforms, locking the tarsometatarsal complex and preventing medial/lateral translation (Figure 1). Thus, dislocation of the metatarsals or cuneiforms typically also involve fracture of the second metatarsal. Additional dynamic stability of the tarsometatarsal joint is offered by the posterior and anterior tibial tendons and peroneal tendons.

All of the bones of the midfoot are attached to their neighbors by ligaments with one exception: there is no ligament connecting the first and second metatarsal. This creates a point of weakness between the first and the other metatarsals. There is an oblique ligament, designated the Lisfranc ligament, which traverses from the plantar-lateral aspect of the medial cuneiform to the plantar-medial aspect of the second metatarsal. Biomechanical studies have shown the Lisfranc ligament to be significantly stronger and stiffer than the plantar and dorsal cuneometatarsal ligaments, making it the main stabilizer of the midfoot.

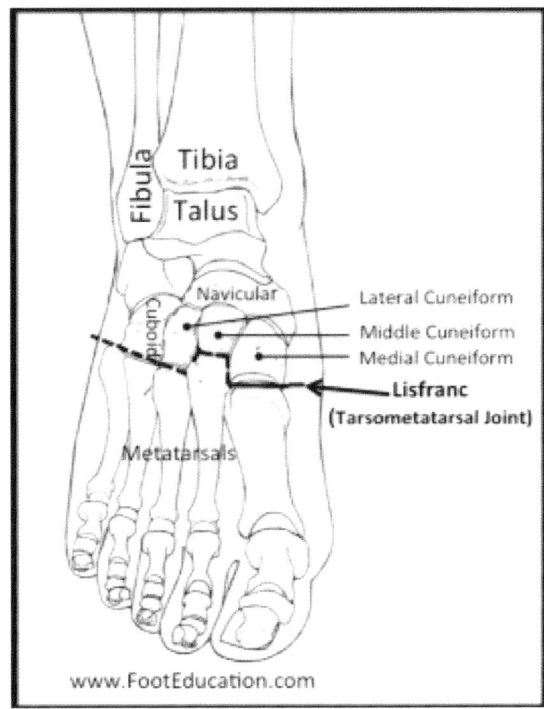

Figure 1: The Lisfranc Joint Complex

PATIENT PRESENTATION

Patients with acute Lisfranc injuries will present with a history of a traumatic injury to the foot. These injuries can be caused by a low-energy injury such as a twisting fall, or by a high-energy injury such as a fall from a height. Sporting activities that require the use of foot straps, such as windsurfing and horse-back riding seem to place people at high risk of this injury. It is also seen more commonly in football players: a force directed down onto the planted foot by a falling player or tackle from behind can lead to hyperplantarflexion at the Lisfranc joint. A similar force is created during high speed motor vehicle collisions, where the foot is often driven into the floorboard (hyperflexing it) as the driver attempts to brake to avoid the crash.

Gross subluxation or lateral deviation of the foot is rare with this injury occurring only in the most severe cases of Lisfranc injuries. As such, pain in the midfoot region, swelling and bruising on the center plantar surface, and pain with weight-bearing may be the only findings that suggest the diagnosis of Lisfranc injuries.

A Lisfranc injury may be stable or unstable. Stable Lisfranc injuries are characterized by a ligamentous injury that is not severe enough to allow the tarsometatarsal joints to displace. Stable Lisfranc injuries typically have no apparent fractures, or fractures that are non-displaced. However, stable Lisfranc injuries still cause significant discomfort because the ligaments of the midfoot are normally subject to marked forces (1-3 times greater than body weight) during normal standing and walking. Therefore, even stable injuries are painful and have a prolonged recovery period. Unstable Lisfranc injuries result in displacement of some or all of the tarsometatarsal joint with associated complete ligament disruption and/or significant fractures of the metatarsal base(s).

OBJECTIVE EVIDENCE

On physical exam, Lisfranc injuries may be manifest as plantar ecchymosis – bruising along the sole of the midfoot (Figure 2). A diminished dorsalis pedis pulse (the artery courses over the proximal head of the second metatarsal) can indicate a more severe dislocation.

Palpation of the foot produces maximum tenderness at the base of the first and second metatarsals. If weight-bearing is even possible, one might see a gap between the big and second toe in the injured foot (the gap sign), as well as a convex bulge at the midfoot on the medial border.

Radiographs should include weight-bearing anteroposterior, lateral views, and 30-degree oblique views. These should be assessed for any fractures, dislocations, or incongruity of the tarsometatarsal joints. Obtaining a comparison image of the other foot is useful to have a reference for normal alignment.

On review of the AP films, the space between the bases of first/second metatarsals and between the medial/middle cuneiforms should be closely examined. Alignment of the medial border of the second metatarsal/middle cuneiform and the medial border of the first metatarsal/medial cuneiform should also be assessed (Figure 3). On lateral films, the superior border of the metatarsal base is normally aligned with the superior border of its corresponding tarsal, but when injured, the metatarsals may sometimes be shifted dorsally or plantar relative to their respective tarsal bone.

A radiographic finding pathognomonic of a Lisfranc injury is the "fleck sign" (Figure 4). This is produced by a bony fragment avulsed at the attachment of the Lisfranc ligament and lying between the bases of the first and second metatarsals.

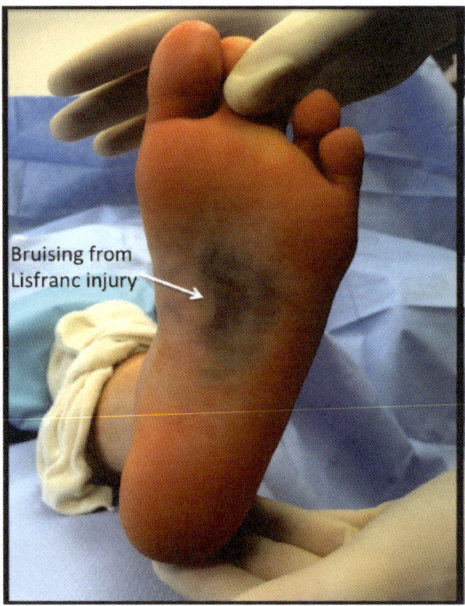

Figure 2: Plantar Ecchymosis following a Lisfranc Injury

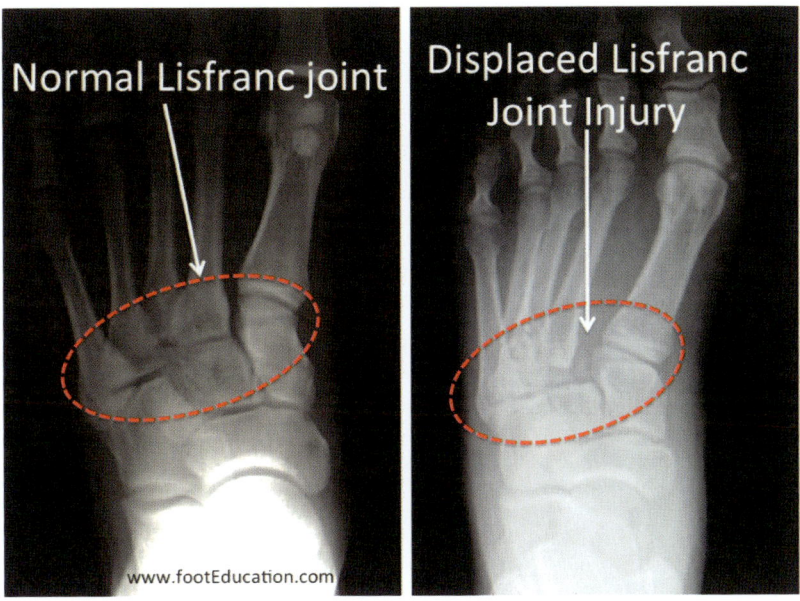

Figure 3: Lisfranc AP X-rays. Anteroposterior radiograph demonstrating: Normal midfoot alignment (Left), Fracture of the second metatarsal and subluxation of the Lisfranc joint (Right).

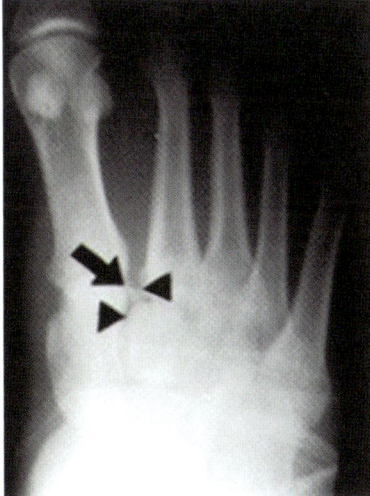

Figure 4: Fleck Sign

EPIDEMIOLOGY

Lisfranc joint injuries are rare and frequently misdiagnosed. The incidence of Lisfranc fracture-dislocations are 1 in 55,000 persons per year, accounting for less than 1% of all fractures. Furthermore, as many as 20% of Lisfranc injuries are missed on initial radiographs.

DIFFERENTIAL DIAGNOSIS

If there is concern about a midfoot injury, a navicular fracture, rupture or avulsion of the posterior tibial tendon should be considered. It is also possible to separate, or avulse, an accessory navicular (an "extra bone" seen in about 10% of the population), creating a painful prominence.

RED FLAGS

Midfoot pain after trauma is a red flag symptom. It is often a manifestation of a Lisfranc injury. Pain and swelling in the midfoot following an acute injury should be considered a Lisfranc injury until proven otherwise.

TREATMENT OPTIONS AND OUTCOMES

For stable injuries, immobilization is recommended. Patients are usually asked to be non-weight bearing or limited weight-bearing through the heel for 6 weeks. After 6 weeks, the patient can gradually increase activity levels. However, full recovery can take several months as the midfoot ligaments must heal enough to stabilize the midfoot joints during gait. An early accurate diagnosis of a Lisfranc injury is important for good functional outcome and proper management. An accurate outline of the prognosis is important for patients. Unlike an ankle sprain, a midfoot sprain (Lisfranc injury) will often take many months to fully recover and may be associated with residual symptoms.

Operative Treatment of Lisfranc Injuries

Surgery should be considered in unstable injuries. Surgery should be undertaken either immediately (before significant swelling occurs) or after allowing the swelling to settle – approximately 7 to 10 days after injury. Surgical fixation allows the bones and ligaments to be held in place for proper healing. This procedure involves reducing and fixing each affected tarsometatarsal joint with screws and/or a plate (Figure 5). The first metatarsal-medial cuneiform articulation is reduced and stabilized first, as this maneuver often reduces the second metatarsal-middle cuneiform joint (Lisfranc complex) as well. Reduction of the fracture-dislocation of the second metatarsal is essential, and firm opposition of the lateral border of the medial cuneiform to the second metatarsal allows for healing of Lisfranc's ligament. A subsequent surgery to remove the hardware may be necessary.

If the diagnosis is delayed or the injury is associated with a complete disruption of the midfoot ligaments, arthrodesis (fusion of the bones making up the involved 1st-3rd tarsometatarsal joints) may be required to successfully address a Lisfranc injury. An arthrodesis (fusion) eliminates motion in the affected joint completely. Prospective randomized studies seem to suggest primary arthrodesis may result in better short-term and medium-term outcomes for unstable displaced Lisfranc injuries when compared to fixation. The rate of secondary surgeries (planned and unplanned, including hardware removal and salvage arthrodesis) are reduced with primary arthrodesis. However, it is unclear whether fixation offers better long-term functional result.

After surgery, a period of non-weight-bearing for 6 to 8 weeks is recommended. Weight-bearing is started while the patient is in the boot if the x-rays look appropriate after 6 to 8 weeks. A return to impact activities, such as running and jumping, may take six months or more. It takes at least a year and often much longer to achieve maximal improvement – and indeed some athletes never return to their pre-injury levels of sport after these injuries.

Even with excellent surgical reduction and fixation, midfoot arthritis may occur from damage to the cartilage. This can lead to chronic midfoot pain and may require fusion in the future. Post-traumatic arthritis is the most common complication (occurring in up to 50% of cases) of Lisfranc joint injury, which is related to the degree of comminution of the articular surface.

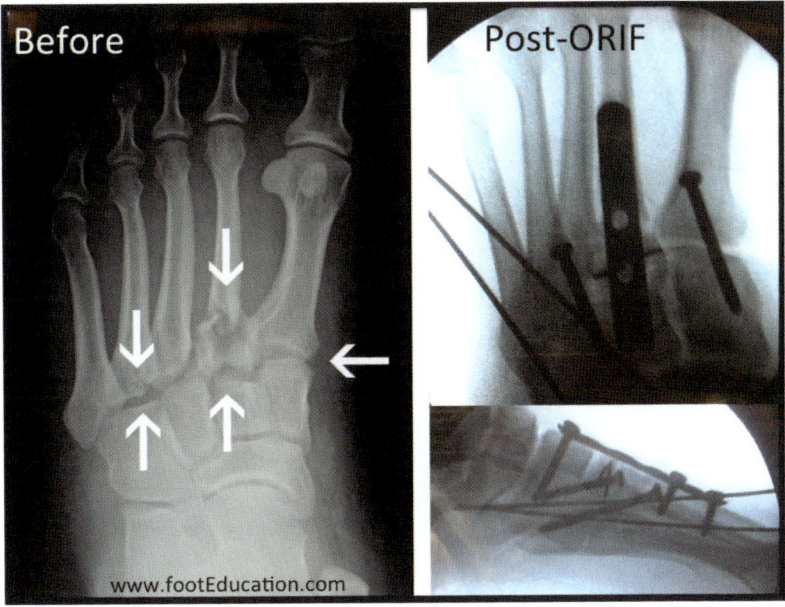

Figure 5: Lisfranc Injury Treated with ORIF

Common sequelae of Lisfranc injuries include late midfoot collapse (flatfoot deformity), metatarsalgia, posttraumatic arthritis. Post-traumatic midfoot arthritis and flatfoot deformity can occur in up to 50% of cases.

MISCELLANY

Jacques Lisfranc de St. Martin (1787-1847), a French Napoleonic-era physician, initially lent his name only to an operation: the Lisfranc amputation. This was an amputation of the foot at the tarsometatarsal joint, used to treat gangrene of the forefoot. Soldiers who fell from a horse with their feet stuck in the stirrup and injured their tarsometatarsal joint frequently, in turn, disrupted the dorsalis pedis artery. Although better diagnosis and treatment has obviated the need for amputations following tarsometatarsal joint injury, the surgeon's name has remained linked to the tarsometatarsal joint. (Lisfranc amputations are still performed for gangrene, though these days the etiology is more commonly diabetes-related vascular disease.)

KEY TERMS

Lisfranc injury, Lisfranc ligament, fleck sign, plantar ecchymosis, midfoot arthritis, Lisfranc open reduction internal fixation (ORIF)

SKILLS

Recognize the physical exam signs of a Lisfranc injury. Assess foot radiographs for the integrity of the tarsometatarsal joint.

CHAPTER 18.

HINDFOOT FRACTURES

DESCRIPTION

Fractures of the calcaneus and talus, collectively termed "hindfoot fractures" are typically caused by high-impact forces like falls or motor vehicle accidents. Calcaneus fractures are more common. Talus fractures though less common, are often associated with greater morbidity owing to the bone's tenuous blood supply of the talus and the associated problem of osteonecrosis. Hindfoot fractures are caused by axial load, and therefore can be seen in conjunction with more proximal injuries, such as fracture of the pelvis or spine – so much so, that a calcaneus fracture should prompt a detailed exam of the spine and pelvis.

STRUCTURE AND FUNCTION

The hindfoot begins at the talocrural (ankle) joint and ends at the calcaneocuboid joint (Figure 1). The bones of the hindfoot are the talus (lower bone of the ankle joint) and the calcaneus (heel bone). The articulation between the talus and calcaneus is called the subtalar joint. The talus does not sit directly on top of the center of the calcaneus, but rather toward the medial-superior edge of the calcaneus (Figure 2).

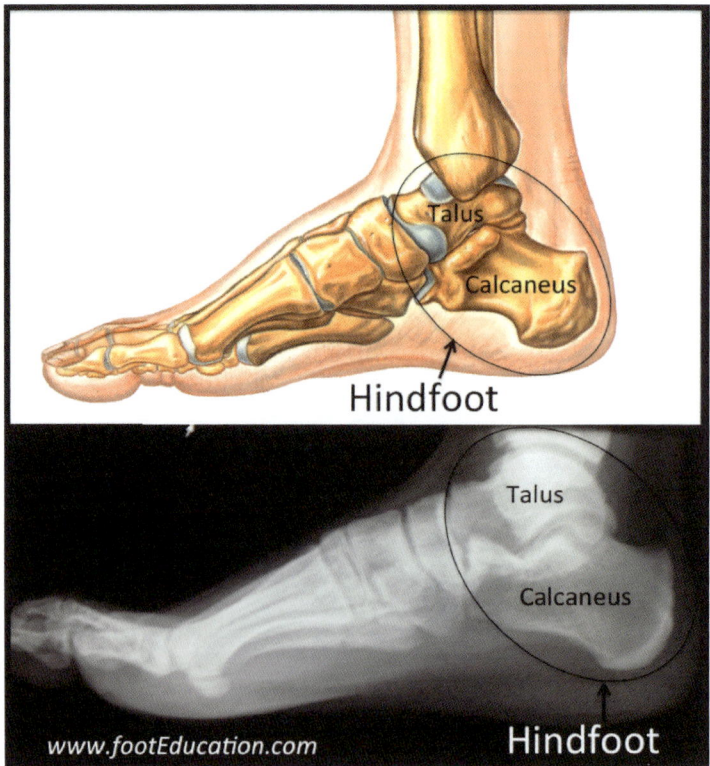

Figure 1: Hindfoot Anatomy

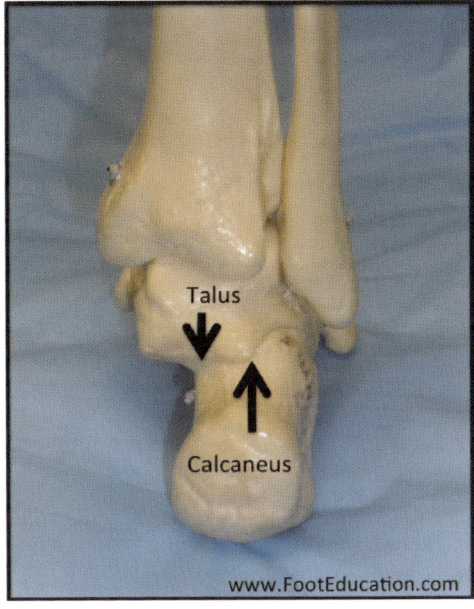

Figure 2: Lateral Offset of Calcaneus on Talus

The hindfoot functions to bear and distribute weight to the foot while standing, and to permit complex foot movements in coordination with the ankle joint, especially inversion/eversion and axial rotation.

The talus has a complex architecture, enabling it to function as a "ball-joint" between the leg and the foot. The talus can be divided into three anatomical regions: the head, neck, and body (Figure 3). The head articulates with the navicular anteriorly (talonavicular joint). The neck connects the body and head and is the most commonly fractured part of the talus.

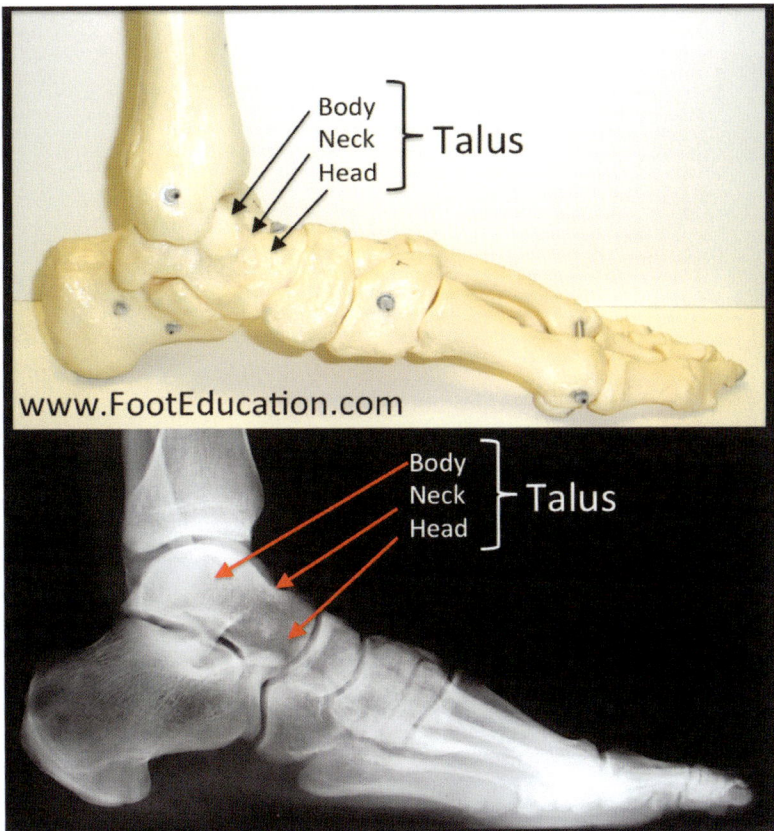

Figure 3: Talar Anatomy

The vascular supply to the body enters at the neck. As such, a fracture of the talar neck may impede perfusion of the talar body. Without perfusion, the bone may die (ie, undergo avascular necrosis). The talar body articulates with the calcaneus inferiorly (subtalar joint) at three separate articular surfaces: anterior, middle, and posterior. There is a small space between these three articulations known as the tarsal sinus.

Motions near the hindfoot include plantarflexion/dorsiflexion at the ankle joint. There is a complex set of motions as the foot moves under the talus at the subtalar and talonavicualr joints. The main elements of this motion is pronation/supination at the subtalar joint; and dorsiflexion and eversion at the talonavicular joint.

Nearly 70% of the talus is covered by articular cartilage. Unlike the calcaneus, which has many insertions and origins of muscles, the talus does not have any muscular attachments. The blood supply to the bone is therefore limited to a "vascular sling" around the talar neck comprising the artery of the tarsal canal (a branch of the posterior tibial artery that supplies the body) and the artery of the tarsal sinus (supplied by branches of the anterior tibial and peroneal arteries to supply the head and neck). This limited blood supply makes the talus prone to delayed healing and avascular necrosis.

The os trigonum is an accessory bone that develops posterior to the talus (Figure 4). It is present in 2.5-14% of people and is bilateral in 60% of these people. For those unfamiliar with this anatomic variation it can be mistaken on x-ray as a fracture of the posterior talus.

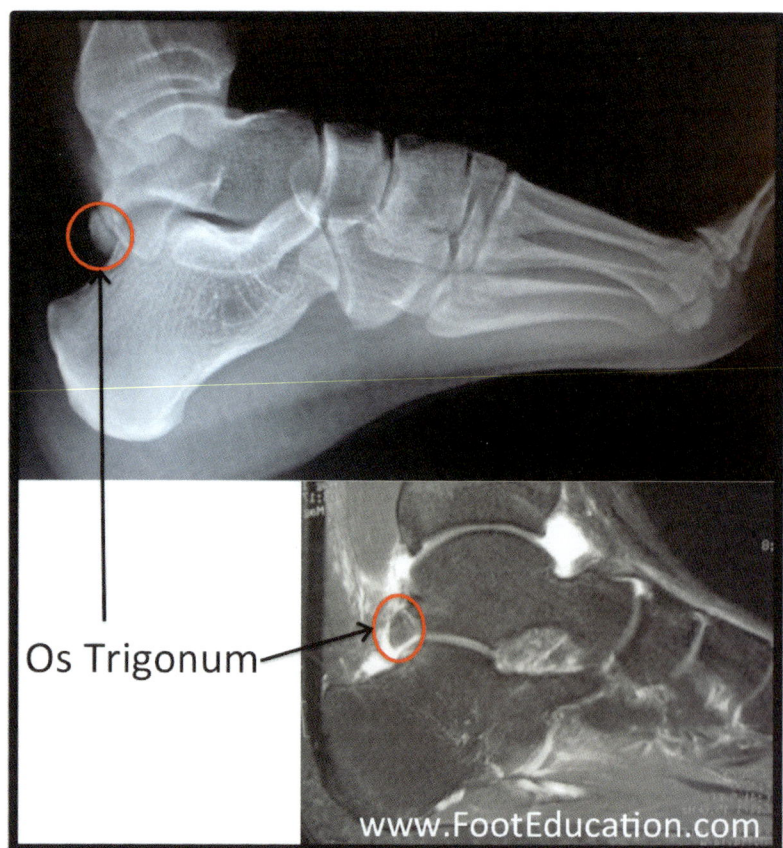

Figure 4: Os Trigonum (circled in red) on Plain Ankle X-ray (Top) and MRI (Bottom).

The calcaneus articulates with the cuboid anteriorly, but its major articulation is with the talus above it. The calcaneus has three anatomic regions: the anterior process, the body, and the posterior tuberosity. The Achilles tendon inserts at the calcaneal tuberosity on the posterior side of the calcaneus. Near the medial talar articulation is the sustentaculum tali (a horizontal shelf of bone). The calcaneus is likened to a "hard-boiled egg" because its outer cortex is thin and surrounds the softer inner cancellous bone. If damaged, the outer cortex can collapse leading to severe comminution of the underlying cancellous bone.

PATIENT PRESENTATION

Patients with a traumatic fracture involving the hindfoot (talus and/or calcaneus) will have a history of an acute injury. Commonly the injury mechanism is an axial load such as occurs in a fall from a height or a motor vehicle accident. Patients will present with significant swelling and pain. It can be difficult to distinguish a fracture from a sprain with an acutely swollen ankle. A laceration, blood, or puncture wound, often on the medial aspect of the foot, is indicative of an open fracture.

Inability to bear weight is a common sign of hindfoot fractures. Redness, hematoma, and fracture blisters may be present near the heel. Fracture blisters occur when excessive swelling causes the layers of the skin to shear leading to localized blisters. A "Mondor sign" is a hematoma extending distally along the sole of the foot – it is a common finding in patients with a calcaneus fracture (Figure 5).

Hindfoot fractures are often accompanied by other injuries because the extent of axial loading necessary to cause a hindfoot fracture is likely to cause other problems too. Fractures and dislocations of the ankle joint may occur in these settings. Additionally, lumbar spine fractures are seen in 10% of patients with calcaneus fractures.

It is important to assess soft tissue damage in addition to the fracture, as the extent of soft tissue damage will dictate the timing of definitive treatment as well as the prognosis. A comprehensive neurological exam should be performed to look for motor or sensory nerve injury. Anterior and posterior tibial pulses and distal capillary refill should be examined via palpation and/or Doppler to assess for any vascular deficits.

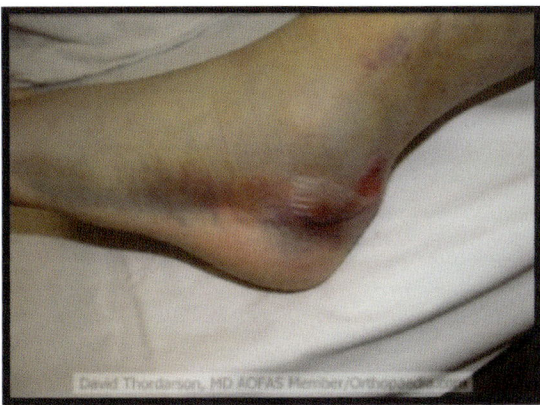

Figure 5: Gross Appearance of a Closed Calcaneal Fracture. Note swelling, bruising, and blister formation along the lateral hindfoot (Mondor sign). Courtesy of David Thordarson MD

OBJECTIVE EVIDENCE

Talar Fractures

The presence and location of talar fractures should be evident on plain films, but the talus may be obscured by the ankle mortise, calcaneus, and midfoot.

Talar neck fractures, caused by excessive dorsiflexion of the foot against the distal tibia, comprise half of all talus fractures (Figure 6). They are classified, with increasing severity, as nondisplaced; displaced but with an intact ankle joint; and displaced with subluxation/dislocation of both the subtalar joint and ankles joints. A fourth category is designated in there is disruption of the talonavicular joint as well.

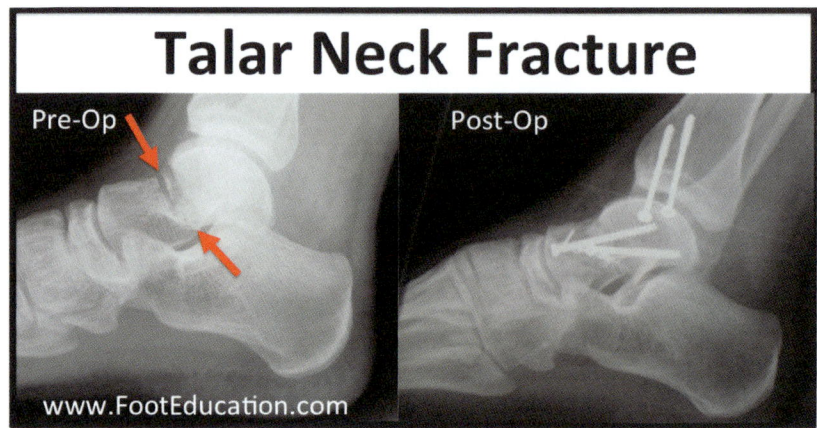

Figure 6: Talar Neck Fracture Pre and Post-Op X-Rays

The second most common site of talus fracture is the lateral process – approximately one-quarter of talus fractures occur here (Figure 7). These often occur following axial compression, dorsiflexion, and eversion. They are common in snowboarders.

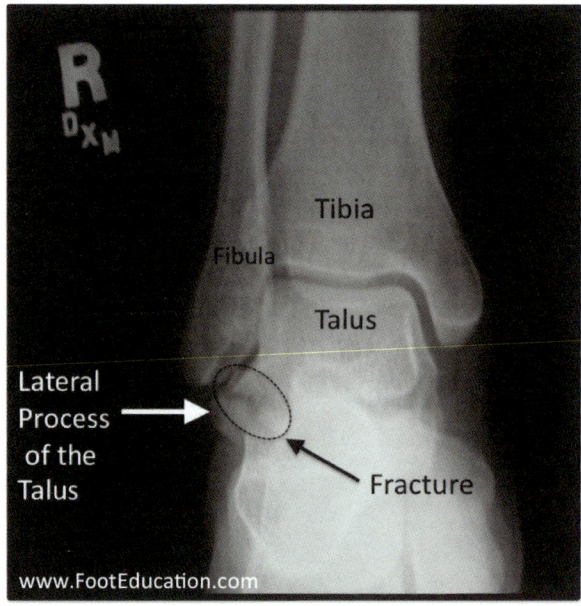

Figure 7: Talar Lateral Process Fracture

Fractures of the talar head, body, and posterior process are less common.

Calcaneal Fractures

Calcaneus fractures are more common than talus fractures. They are broadly classified according to whether they involve the subtalar articular surface (intra-articular) or not (extra-articular).

Extra-articular fractures represent only 25% of calcaneal fractures. By definition, they do not involve the subtalar joint or its articular surfaces. Extra-articular fractures typically affect the anterior process, calcaneal tuberosity, calcaneal body, and sustentaculum. Intra-articular fractures are more common (Figure 8). They are also more challenging to treat.

An ankle (anterior-posterior, mortise, and lateral) and foot (AP, oblique, and lateral) x-rays series should be taken. Two angles on the lateral x-ray can be helpful in assessing calcaneus fractures. Bohler's angle is formed from two lines: (1) a line drawn from the superior point of the posterior calcaneal tuberosity to the highest midpoint of the posterior articular facet, and (2) the highest midpoint of the posterior articular facet to the anterior process (Figure 8). This angle should be 20-40 degrees – a decrease in Bohler's angle suggests a depressed fracture of the posterior facet. The Angle of Gissane (Figure 9) is formed from the downward slope of the posterior facet and the upward slope directed anteriorly. This angle should be 100-130 degrees – an increase suggests a fracture of the posterior subtalar articular surface.

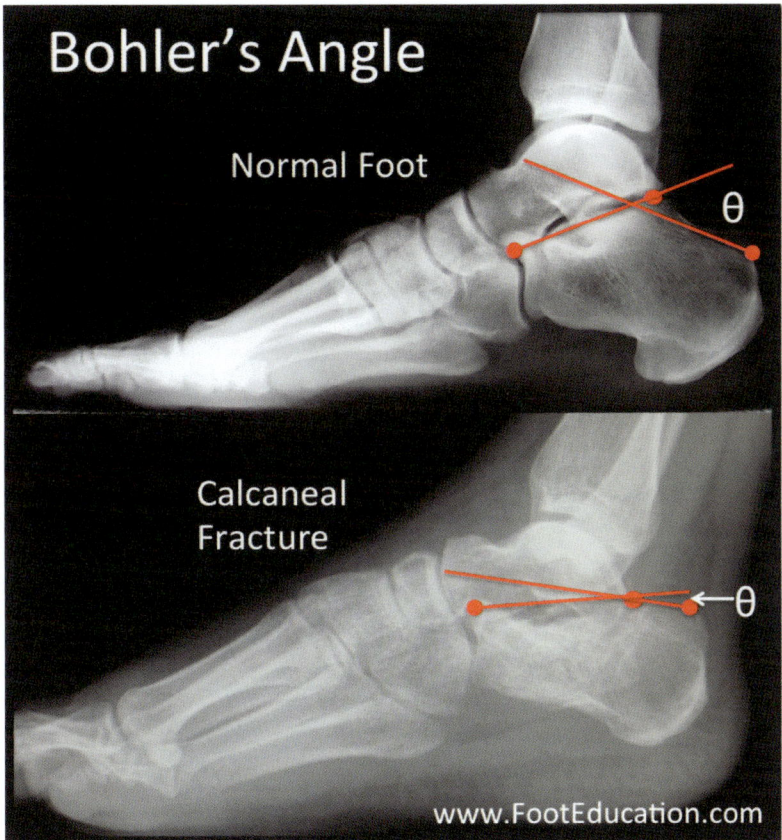

Figure 8: Normal (Top) and Abnormal (Bottom) Bohler's Angle on Lateral Foot X-Ray.

A depressed calcaneal fracture leads to a lower Bohler's angle (<20 degrees)

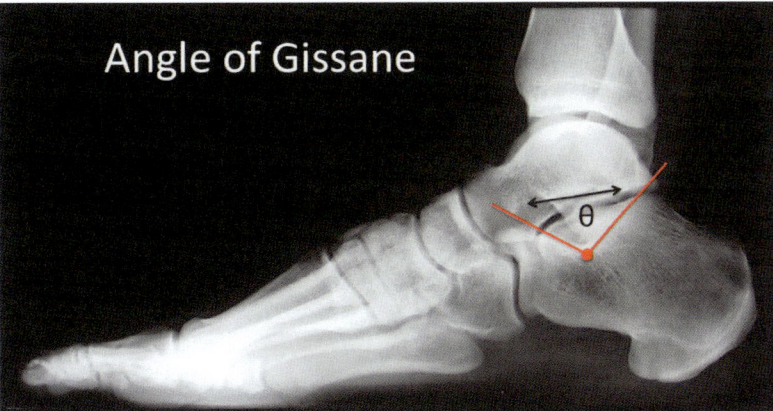

Figure 9: Angle of Gissane (Normal)

"Hawkins sign," namely a radiolucent line in the subchondral talus (patchy subchondral osteopenia) several weeks following injury on the AP or mortise views of the ankle, is a radiographic indicator of revascularization and absence of avascular necrosis. The radiolucency is the result of bone resorption and is a good sign – it indicates that the bone retained its blood supply.

CT imaging is routinely performed to assess the fracture pattern, degree of displacement, and involvement of articular surfaces since radiographic imaging does not provide sufficient resolution to visualize the articular fragments. Sagittal, coronal, and transverse CT scans are especially helpful for the decisions to perform surgery as well as intra-operative decision-making about technique and needed implants.

MRI is mostly used to detect and quantify the degree of avascular necrosis of talar fractures. It is also used to diagnose osteochondral lesions of the talus.

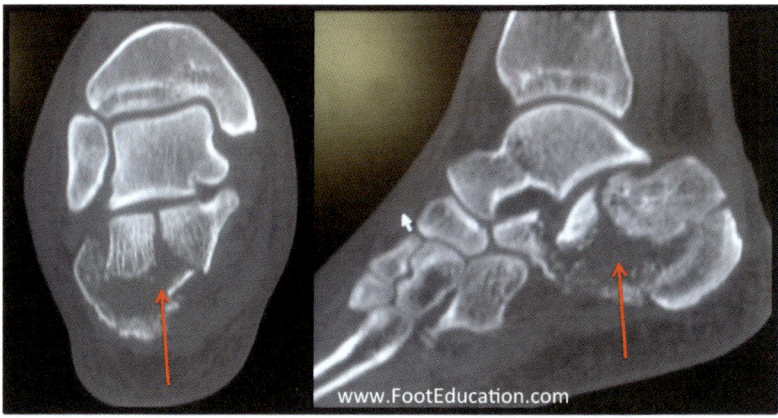

Figure 10: CT Scan of Calcaneus Fracture: Coronal View (left), Sagittal View (right)

EPIDEMIOLOGY

Calcaneus fractures comprise 2% of all fractures and 60% of tarsal fractures. The annual incidence is approximately 12 per 100,000 per year, significantly less than ankle fractures (187 per 100,000) which may present similarly. Calcaneus fractures occur 2.4 times more often in males and most often affect men in their 20's. 72% of calcaneal fractures are due to falls from a height and 19% occur in the workplace. A small minority of calcaneus fractures may be non-traumatic stress fractures due to repetitive axial loading, as seen in military personnel or long-distance runners. Ten percent of calcaneus fractures are bilateral. Ten percent will have associated thoracolumbar spine injuries and another 10% will have a hip fracture.

Talus fractures are the second most common fractured bone in the foot but are rarer than calcaneus fractures, comprising only 0.1-0.9% of all fractures. The most common site of talus fractures is at the talar neck followed by the lateral process. Talus fractures are significant because of their potential for long-term morbidity and complications.

Open fractures occur in approximately 20% of calcaneus and talus fractures.

DIFFERENTIAL DIAGNOSIS

High-energy impact is necessary to cause hindfoot fractures and this may cause other injuries to the lower limb. These associated injuries can include ankle sprains, ankle fractures, talus dislocations, tibial and fibular fractures, pilon fractures, hip fractures, and injuries to the other tarsal and metatarsal bones. In fact, one-quarter of calcaneal fractures are accompanied by other lower limb injuries. A high-energy axial load can also cause injuries outside the lower limb. One of the most common injuries is a thoracolumbar spine fracture, which occurs in 10% of patients with calcaneal fractures.

RED FLAGS

Hindfoot fractures can be missed in patients who have sustained polytraumatic injuries. Thus an axial load mechanism should be a "red flag" suggesting the presence of a hindfoot fracture, and the presence of such a fracture in one limb should prompt close evaluation of the contralateral side (as it may have been subjected to the same axial load) as well as the spine and pelvis.

A missed hindfoot fracture should also be suspected if a diagnosed ankle sprain does not improve with routine treatment. Subtle hindfoot fractures such as a fracture of the anterior process of the calcaneus can be caused by the same inversion mechanism that causes sprains, and therefore can be easily misdiagnosed as ankle sprains.

Tenting of the skin with a fracture is a worrisome sign indicative of potential skin necrosis.

TREATMENT OPTIONS AND OUTCOMES

Initial treatment of hindfoot fractures should focus on reducing swelling and addressing any open wounds. After the fracture pattern has been identified, definitive treatment can begin.

Definitive treatment for hindfoot fractures can be operative or non-operative depending on the part of the bone fractured, the severity of the fracture, and the patient's risk factors. Non-operative treatment generally involves relative immobilization and no weight-bearing for 6 to 12 weeks followed by progressive weight-bearing. Gentle early ankle and hindfoot range of motion exercises are an important element of non-operative treatment for calcaneal fractures and other stable hindfoot injuries. An attempt to move the hindfoot relatively early in the recovery period will help minimize residual hindfoot stiffness – although some stiffness is inevitable.

Operative treatment generally involves open reduction and internal fixation (ORIF) followed by immobilization, no weight-bearing, and early ROM exercises. There is a window of opportunity for surgery – long enough after the injury such that there is resolution of swelling, yet not too long that too much soft callus has formed.

The risk of complications of talar neck and body fractures is related to the extent of the displacement, degree of damage to the blood supply, and damage to the articular surfaces. A common complication is avascular necrosis of the talar body due to injury to the vascular sling supplying the talus. The risk of avascular necrosis in talar neck fractures is 10% or less if the fracture is not displaced; the risk is close to 100% if there is disruption of subtalar, ankle and talonavicular joints.

Displaced lateral talar process fractures typically have a better outcome than talar neck and body fractures. They are treated by stabilizing the fracture fragment with screws (Figure 11). If the fractured fragment is small or comminuted, it can be removed.

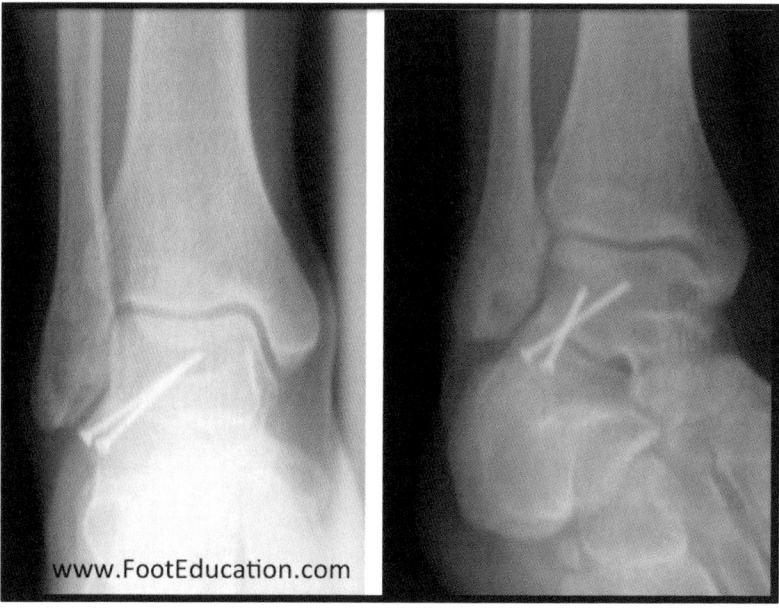

Figure 11: Surgical Fixation of a Lateral Process Fracture of the Talus

Extra-articular calcaneus fractures can generally be treated non-operatively unless the fragments are large. In the case of fractures of the calcaneal tuberosity caused by Achilles tendon avulsion, screw fixation may be required to prevent displacement by the force of the Achilles.

Non-displaced calcaneal fractures are treated non-operatively and either non-operative or surgical fixation may be indicated for displaced calcaneal fractures (Figure 12). Effective surgical treatment of a displaced calcaneal fracture is a highly technical procedure. Surgical fixation has not been shown to be superior to non-operative treatment in multiple comparative studies when considering all patients and reviewing all outcomes. The potential benefits of surgery including better range of motion, improved function, and less posttraumatic subtalar arthritis are offset by the higher wound complication and infection rates in the surgically treated patients. It has been shown that surgical fixation has optimal results in young, female patients who are not receiving worker's compensation. Smokers, diabetics, older patients, patients with vascular disease, and those receiving worker's compensation tend to do less well.

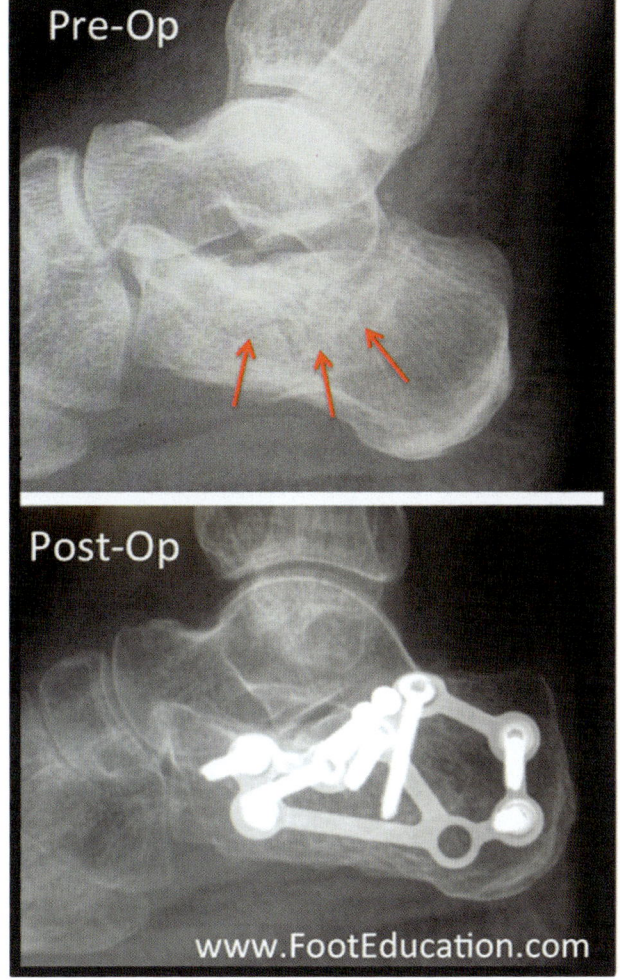

Figure 12: X-Ray of Depressed Calcaneal Fracture Pre and Post ORIF.

RISK FACTORS AND PREVENTION

Because most hindfoot fractures occur in the setting of acute injury, such as falls or motor vehicle accidents, prevention mostly centers on avoiding such accidents. However, certain health conditions can also predispose people to hindfoot fractures. For example, diabetes mellitus and low bone mineral density are major risk factors for hindfoot fractures.

Hindfoot fractures can also be sports-related. Snowboarders are 17 times more likely to sustain fractures to the lateral process of the talus compared to the general population. Additionally, running with minimalist footwear has been implicated in calcaneal stress fractures.

MISCELLANY

Calcaneus fractures are called "lover's fractures" because they are the injury a cheating spouse would sustain if jumping from an upstairs bedroom window to escape trouble.

Talus fractures were historically referred to as "Aviator's astralgus." In the early 20th century, plane crashes at sub-lethal speeds were common, resulting in high-impact injuries to the foot including talus fractures. Nowadays talus fractures are mostly caused by falls and motor vehicle accidents, so this term is mostly obsolete.

KEY TERMS

Talus fracture, Calcaneus fracture, Osteonecrosis, Os trigonum, Mondor sign, Hawkins sign, Bohler's angle, Aviator's astralgus

SKILLS

Develop a differential diagnosis of possible foot injuries resulting from high-energy axial loading such as a fall or motor vehicle accident. Recognize the classic signs, symptoms, and history of hindfoot fractures. Identify and differentiate between calcaneus and talus fractures on plain radiographs. Use radiography to calculate Bohler's and Gissane's angles. Classify calcaneus fractures according to Sanders Classification using coronal CT images. Determine the appropriateness of operative vs. non-operative management depending on whether fractures are displaced and the patients associated risk factors.

CHAPTER 19.

METATARSAL FRACTURES

DESCRIPTION

Metatarsal fractures are common injuries to the foot often sustained with direct blows or twisting forces. Many of these fractures are easy to treat and have a favorable prognosis. However, metatarsal fractures that go on to malunion or nonunion can lead to disabling metatarsalgia or midfoot arthritis. The metatarsals are also subject to stress fractures and can be seen in conjunction with other injuries of the mid-foot.

STRUCTURE AND FUNCTION

The metatarsals are dorsally convex tubular bones of the forefoot consisting of a head, neck, shaft, and base. They are numbered from 1 to 5, medial to lateral or largest to smallest (Figure 1). The base of each metatarsal articulates with one or more of the tarsal bones and the head articulates with the proximal phalanges. The bases of each metatarsal also articulate with each other at the intermetatarsal joints. As a unit, the five metatarsals serve as the major weight-bearing complex of the forefoot. The medial three rays act as a rigid lever to aid in propulsion while the lateral two rays provide some mobility in the sagittal plane to permit accommodation to uneven ground.

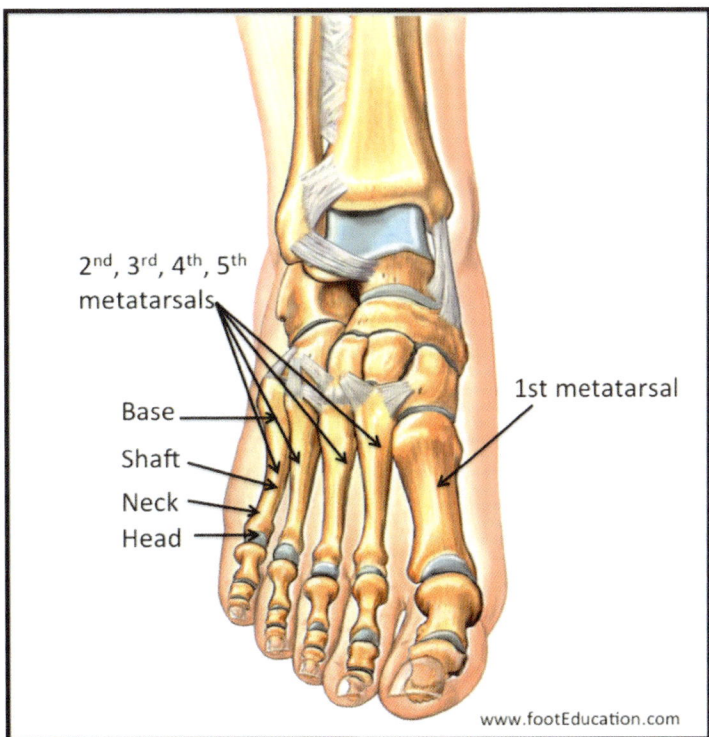

Figure 1. Metatarsal Anatomy

The first metatarsal is larger than the others and most important for weight-bearing and balance; therefore, malunion or malalignment at this location is especially poorly tolerated. There are no interconnecting ligaments between the 1st and 2nd metatarsals, allowing for independent motion.

The second, third and fourth metatarsals are slender and may be sites of stress fracture or acute fractures from twisting mechanisms or a direct blow.

The fifth metatarsal is divided into 3 zones (as shown), numbered 1 to 3 from proximal to distal (Figure 2). Zone 1 is the base of the metatarsal where the peroneus brevis inserts. Avulsion fractures from the pull of this tendon and attached ligaments are characteristic of zone 1. Zone 2 is at the metaphyseal-diaphyseal junction, distal to the cancellous (styloid) tuberosity. Fractures involving Zone 2, called Jones fractures, are particularly susceptible to nonunion and malunion because this region of the bone has a tenuous blood supply. Many of these Jones-type fractures are stress-type fractures caused directly or indirectly by repetitive loading to this area. Zone 3 is the diaphysis and fractures are most commonly trauma or rotational injuries leading to spiral fractures.

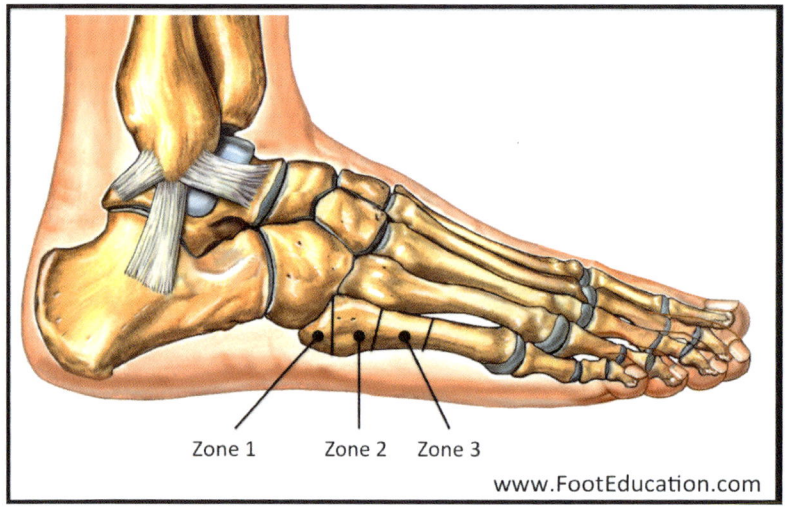

Figure 2. The Zones of 5th Metatarsal. This seemingly arbitrary division is clinically important: fractures in each zone have distinct prognoses and treatment needs.

PATIENT PRESENTATION

Most metatarsal fractures result from an acute injury, although chronic stress fractures and neuropathic related metatarsal fractures do occur. Patients with an acute metatarsal fracture present with pain, swelling, ecchymosis, and tenderness to palpation in the forefoot – along with difficulty bearing weight. Except with major trauma gross deformities are rarely seen.

A history of direct impact suggests a transverse or comminuted fracture of the shaft, while a twisting-type injury typically causes an oblique or spiral fracture pattern.

A physical exam should be performed with specific attention paid to the main areas of pain, which usually correlates to the site of injury. The relative position of the metatarsal heads should be assessed to rule out malposition and other deformities. Gently applying an axial load to the metatarsal head will create pain if that metatarsal is fractured and this may help differentiate a fracture from a soft-tissue injury on clinical exam. A neurovascular examination should be performed to assess for any loss or altered sensation and review the vascularity of the foot and the toes.

OBJECTIVE EVIDENCE

Radiographs in the anteroposterior (AP), oblique, and lateral planes should be obtained (Figure 3). The films should include the entire foot to rule out associated injuries that may require treatment.

The lateral view is important for judging sagittal plane displacement of the metatarsal heads, and the oblique view can help detect minimally displaced fractures.

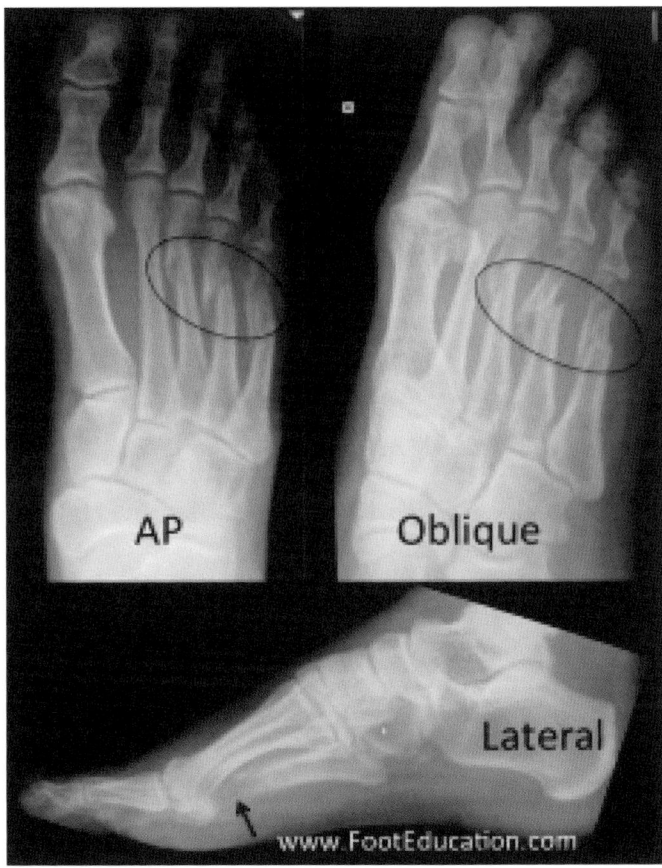

Figure 3: Metatarsal Fractures seen on X-Rays (AP, Oblique, and Lateral) of the Foot

Dancer's Fractures (Avulsion fracture of the base of the 5th metatarsal)

Avulsion fractures occur at the base of the fifth metatarsal, in Zone 1 where the peroneus brevis and plantar fascia insert (Figure 4). These fractures occur during forced inversion of the foot and ankle while plantar flexed. This injury, commonly termed a "Dancer's fracture" (or a pseudo-Jones fracture, a name that should be avoided), can happen after landing awkwardly from a jump or twisting the ankle while running. The ankle passively inverts at the same time the peroneus brevis tendon exerts an eversion force on the metatarsal which is rigidly held by the plantar fascia. A fragment of bone accordingly avulses. There is some confusion and debate about the use of the term *Dancer's Fracture* as it has also been used to describe a spiral fracture of the 5th metatarsal shaft. The original description was apparently coined by legendary orthopaedic surgeon Sir Robert Jones who suffered an avulsion type fracture following an inversion type injury while dancing in 1902. Subsequently a report of spiral 5th metatarsal fractures in dancers was published leading some to describe these injuries as *Dancer's fractures*.

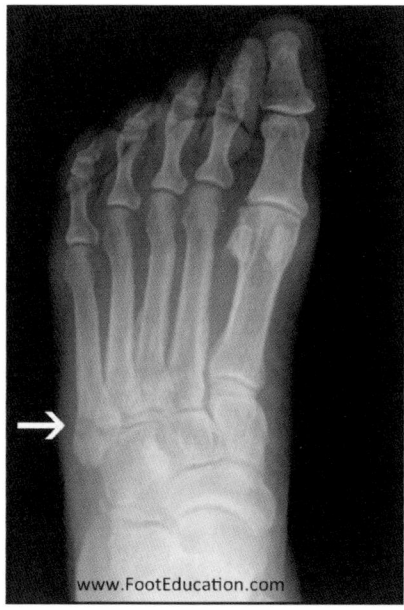

Figure 4. Radiograph of Dancer's Fracture (Avulsion Fracture)- Zone 1 of 5th Metatarsal

Jones Fractures (5th metadiaphyseal stress fractures)

True Jones fractures occur in Zone 2 of the fifth metatarsal (Figure 5). The fracture line extends through the proximal articulation with the fourth metatarsal. This fracture is a result of tensile stress along the lateral border of the metatarsal during adduction or inversion of the forefoot. This type of loading pattern is commonly seen in patients with high arched (subtle cavus) feet. Most Jones fractures are stress fractures related to repetitive loading although there is usually a single precipitating event. An athlete can sustain this injury with a sudden change in direction while the heel is off the ground.

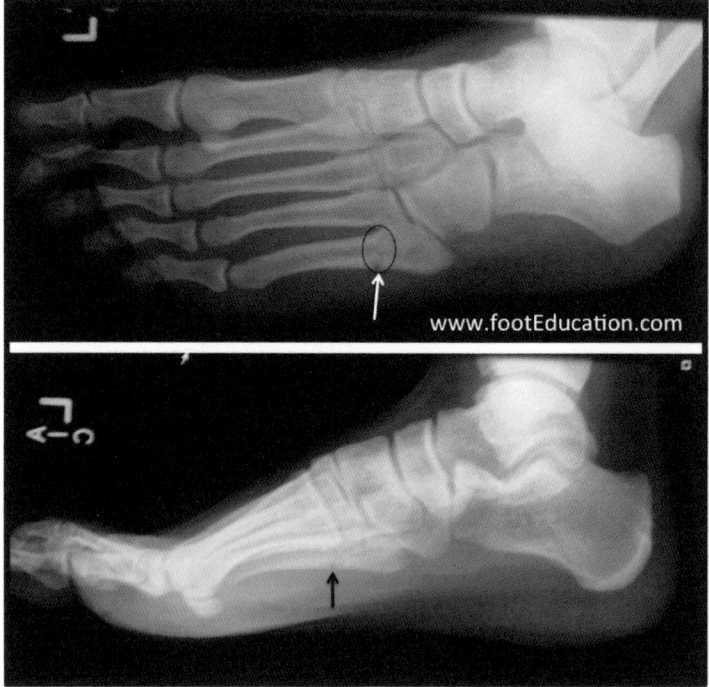

Figure 5: Jones Fracture of the Metadiaphyseal area of the 5th Metatarsal

Metatarsal base fractures and Lisfranc injuries

Fractures of the base of the metatarsal are often associated with disruption of the tarsometatarsal joints – a Lisfranc injury (discussed in its own section). To detect Lisfranc injuries, it is important to carefully examine the radiographs for widening between the 1st and 2nd metatarsal space, fleck fractures at the base of the 1st or 2nd metatarsal, and loss of alignment between the medial edge of the 2nd cuneiform and medial edge of the 2nd metatarsal base. Weight-bearing x-rays are particularly helpful when trying to rule out or assess Lisfranc injuries.

The most common metatarsal shaft fracture pattern is oblique or transverse with minimal displacement. Additional imaging is rarely necessary. However, if there is high suspicion for a Lisfranc fracture, even if the radiographs appear normal, CT scan or MRI can be helpful in identifying these injuries.

Metatarsal stress fractures

Metatarsal stress fractures are rarely visible on plain radiographs until symptoms have been present for 2-6 weeks and a resulting callus appears (Figure 6). Before that, an MRI or technetium bone scan may be necessary to make the diagnosis. Stress fractures involving the second or third metatarsal often occur in the shaft or metatarsal neck region. They commonly occur in individuals who have had a sudden increase in their activity level such as a new military recruit who goes on a long hike. These fractures are also known as "March fractures." Ballet dancers who are up on their toes can get stress fractures at the base of the second metatarsal.

Neuropathic metatarsal fractures

Individuals with abnormal sensation in their feet, such as patients with diabetic neuropathy, can get stress related fractures in their metatarsals. The fifth metatarsal metadiaphyseal area is a common location for a stress fracture (Jones fracture) particularly if the patient has a high arched foot, or an underlying varus alignment of the lower extremity.

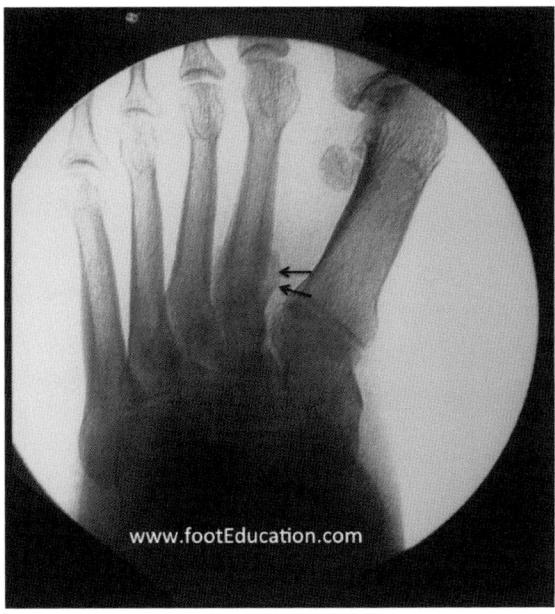

Figure 6: Second Metatarsal Stress Fracture

EPIDEMIOLOGY

Excluding toe fractures, metatarsal fractures are the most common foot fracture. In children, the most commonly injured metatarsals are the first and fifth simply due to their anatomical exposure. In adults, high forces are required to fracture the larger and stronger first metatarsal, so these are much less common. In industrial injuries, the fifth metatarsal is most commonly injured.

DIFFERENTIAL DIAGNOSIS

A metatarsal fracture must be suspected in all patients with direct trauma to the forefoot and pain with ambulation. Maintain a high index of suspicion for an associated Lisfranc injury at the tarsometatarsal joint, especially with the involvement of the proximal first through fourth metatarsals and if the patient has plantar ecchymosis on exam. The metatarsophalangeal joints and phalanges should also be assessed for injury.

RED FLAGS

In some sense, a metatarsal fracture is itself a red flag, calling attention to the need to exclude a more serious injury. In particular, fractures of the 2nd, 3rd or 4th metatarsal should raise suspicion of a ligament (Lisfranc) injury. A 5th metatarsal fracture must be scrutinized to make sure a zone 2 (Jones) fracture (which needs more protection) is identified. A 1st metatarsal fracture must be examined closely to ensure there is no displacement. In short, Lisfranc injuries, zone 2 5th metatarsal fractures, and displaced 1st metatarsal fractures must be detected, and the presence of any fracture near their regions is a red flag alerting the examiner to their possible presence as well.

Pain that persists or even worsens after immobilization may be a sign of a (rare) compartment syndrome of the foot. Late signs include pallor, paresthesias, and tense swelling – but don't wait for them to appear.

Plantar bruising is often indicative of a serious injury such as a Lisfranc injury.

Redness and swelling of the forefoot may indicate a Charcot neuropathic fracture in a patient with loss of sensation.

TREATMENT OPTIONS AND OUTCOMES

The goal of treatment is to restore alignment of the 5 metatarsals to preserve the arches of the foot and allow normal weight distribution over the metatarsal heads.

Management varies widely depending on the location of the injury. Most isolated central (2nd – 4th) metatarsal fractures, as well as non-displaced fractures of the 1st metatarsal, can be treated with a walking boot and progressive weight bearing as tolerated. Displacement of a first metatarsal fracture usually represents an unstable pattern that requires surgical fixation.

Treatment of fifth metatarsal fractures depends on the Zone of injury. Non-displaced and minimally displaced avulsion fractures (Dancer's Fractures or Zone 1) may only require symptomatic therapy with a hard shoe or walking boot until the fracture heals. However, full healing of avulsion-type 5th metatarsal fractures often take 8 weeks or longer.

Jones fractures, those in Zone 2, require at the minimum a non-weight-bearing cast or boot for an extended period (ex. 6 weeks) with a protective stiff soled boot or shoe during a graduated return to weight-bearing for 6 or more weeks thereafter. Immediate surgical fixation of Jones fractures may be offered to speed the rate of healing and lower the incidence of nonunion.

Most metatarsal fractures will go on to heal uneventfully with appropriate treatment, but complications do occur. Malunion, nonunion, or arthritic degeneration of the TMT and MTP joints can lead to metatarsalgia and significant disability, especially in the 1st metatarsal. In addition, malunion can cause plantar keratoses (painful callus) from significant plantar deviation of the metatarsal heads and dorsal keratoses from uncorrected dorsal angulation. Like with all fractures, insuring adequate levels of Vitamin D prevents delays and non-unions of fracture healing.

Non-surgical treatment is advocated in patients with vascular comprise and neuropathy, as risk of infection and nonunion is elevated. Patients with diabetes are still candidates for fixation providing they have good vascular supply and protective sensation to extremities.

RISK FACTORS AND PREVENTION

Not much can be done to prevent an injury to the metatarsal if a large force is applied to the foot in a traumatic incident. However, wearing appropriate protective footwear can be markedly beneficial.

MISCELLANY

An avulsion fracture is fleck of bone pulled off by a ligament or tendon; it is similar to the sliver of paint that may be pulled off a wall when a piece of tape adherent to the wall is removed with sudden force.

The 5th metatarsal growth plate is unusual in that it is at the base of the bone and oriented longitudinally. In children, a fracture needs to be differentiated from a symptomatic secondary ossification center.

KEY TERMS

Metatarsal fracture, Dancer's fracture, Lisfranc joint, Jones fracture, metatarsalgia

SKILLS

Be able to pinpoint fracture site by palpation along each metatarsal. Differentiate soft tissue injury from fracture by gently applying an axial loading to the metatarsal head. Correctly interpret radiographic findings and classify the different types of fractures. Be able to apply a cast or splint the foot.

CHAPTER 20.

STRESS FRACTURES OF THE FOOT

DESCRIPTION

Bone can strengthen over time in response to loading, the same way that, conversely, astronauts lose bone mass when the stress of gravity and walking is removed. Stress fractures occur when a cycle of repetitive forces, none on their own sufficient to cause injury, is applied such that these forces exceed the bone's ability to adapt and cumulatively damage the bone. In cases where the bone is entirely healthy, and the cause is simply too many cycles of load, the injury is denoted as a fatigue or stress fracture. Separately, fractures can also occur in bone that is not healthy, such as in the setting of osteoporosis, and does not stand up to even few cycles of repetitive forces. These are called insufficiency fractures. Repetitive activities such as walking, running and jumping can subject the bones of the foot to large forces that potentially lead to stress fractures, especially if these activities are started abruptly and without a ramp up period that allows the bone to effectively adapt. These injuries are commonly seen in the 2nd or 3rd metatarsal neck region, the base of 5th metatarsal (Jones Fracture), the sesamoid bones of the great toe, the navicular bone, or the calcaneus tuberosity.

STRUCTURE AND FUNCTION

Bone is built to withstand load. Of course, a sufficiently high load applied at one time can cause bone to break. When a sudden injury generates a load higher than the bone's strength, the bone will fracture. Bones can also be broken by cyclical application of subcritical loads, loads which do not cause damage if applied only a limited number of times. However, if too many cycles of such load are applied, or are applied quicker than the bone is able to adapt, stress fractures may ensue.

Repetitive application of a subcritical force causes microscopic damage to the bone. This damage is not a problem so long as the bone remodeling cycle (osteoclasts remove the damaged tissue and osteoblasts synthesize a healthy replacement) can maintain the structural integrity of the bone. There are, however, two instances where cyclical loads do lead to clinical problems. The first is when the bone metabolism is normal, yet the number of cycles is just too high for it to effectively adapt. Structural failure in the setting of normal bone remodeling that is unable to match the demands of high cycles of subcritical load is called a *fatigue fracture*. The second type of stress fracture is an *insufficiency fracture*. It occurs when the bone itself is abnormal, as in osteoporosis, and the cycle of loading would otherwise not have led to a fracture.

Initially in a stress fracture, the gross contour of the bone is normal and the damage is internal. This is sometimes described as a stress reaction. When internal damage accumulates the macroscopic architecture may fail and the bone may overtly fracture into two or more pieces. This is analogous to how paper clips are broken, wherein repetitive small loads are applied by bending the clip back and forth until enough damage accumulates, and the clip is broken in two.

Stress fractures of the feet occur in those bones, and often in the specific locations within those bones that are subjected to the highest repetitive loads. Each person's foot absorbs force in a slightly different manner predicated by that person's foot shape, alignment, foot stiffness, and gait pattern. Therefore, it is common for each foot to be disproportionally exposed to increased load in specific areas.

In certain foot shapes (typically flatfeet) the necks of the 2nd and 3rd metatarsals are subject to increased bending forces with walking. Thus, too much walking, especially with too little rest to allow repair, can cause stress fractures in these regions. This has been seen commonly in military recruits subject to long hikes with heavy backpacks, and therefore often called "march fractures."

In patients with a high arched foot, which disproportionately tips the foot onto its lateral margin, running and sporting activities may subject the base of the 5th metatarsal to overload precipitating a stress fracture. These are frequently referred to as "Jones' fractures" when they occur in the proximal metaphyseal/diaphyseal junction of the 5th metatarsal. This occurs because the high arch foot tends to be a stiffer foot and the heel tilts inward, shifting pressure onto the lateral border of the foot. These fractures may also be precipitated by an acute injury.

The navicular bone, too, is a site of stress fractures especially if the patient has a stiff, high arched foot, a relatively long second metatarsal, and participates in activities that involve dynamic repetitive loading through the forefoot such as sprinting. The mechanism of injury is felt to be repetitive loading through the second metatarsal and middle cuneiform into the navicular.

The sesamoid bones beneath the great toe can develop stress fractures, as found in patients who suddenly increase in running distance. The sesamoids see increased stress with push off activities involved in sprinting or jumping.

The calcaneal tuberosity can also develop stress fractures, usually in response to the repetitive heel strike inherent to some runners. This becomes especially true with sudden increase in mileage.

PATIENT PRESENTATION

Patients with stress fractures will usually report focal aching in the affected area. They may give a history of an increase in their normal activity level. This pain typically increases with activity and decreases with rest. They may have a history of a condition that predisposes them to weaker bones such as osteoporosis (weak thin bone), amenorrhea (loss of normal menstrual cycle), or a history of smoking. Among young female athletes, the "female athletic triad" of an eating disorder, amenorrhea, and low bone density deserves special mention, wherein the presence of 2-3 components of the triad can potentiate stress fractures.

Stress fractures involving the lesser metatarsal bones (typically 2nd or 3rd) will often present with pain and swelling near the metatarsal neck, distally. Occasionally, high-level ballet and modern dancers will generate stress fractures at the base of the metatarsal near the midfoot. The foot type, in general, may be flat, often with a long second and possibly third ray. Early in the condition patients usually can walk without a limp.

Individuals who suffer a Jones' fracture will initially report a dull aching pain on the outside of the midfoot. Patients often persist in their activities despite the pain until there is an overt failure of the bone. At that point they will have difficulty bearing weight and may walk with a pronounced limp.

Patients who develop navicular stress fractures will present with a chronic medial or central mid-foot ache. Although anyone can get a navicular stress fracture, the most common presentation is among athletes. The symptoms of a navicular stress fracture are often generalized to the mid-foot, and the relatively nonspecific location of the symptoms may make this condition difficult to diagnose.

Sesamoid stress fractures do occur, with the caution that in many instances "fracture" of the sesamoid is actually a normal bipartite sesamoid with superimposed sesamoiditis. The pain is usually isolated to under the great toe region.

Calcaneal stress fractures are often in runners and present with heel pain, often after an increase in their training regimen. A calcaneal squeeze test, wherein pain is generated by compressing the calcaneal tuberosity between both thenar eminences, can differentiate this condition from other conditions that often present in runners, such as plantar fasciitis or Achilles tendinitis.

OBJECTIVE EVIDENCE

A good history and physical examination may suggest a stress fracture; however, imaging studies are required to definitively diagnose a stress fracture in the foot. Plain x-rays may be diagnostic, although stress fractures often will not show up on x-rays unless there is enough structural failure of the bone to generate an overt crack, or a healing callus response is found – often weeks after the original stress fracture.

An MRI can demonstrate a stress fracture earlier due to its ability to detect reactive edema in the surrounding bones. Bone scans can also be positive, though their use has diminished with the ubiquitous availability of MRI. A normal MRI or bone scan effectively excludes the diagnosis of a stress fracture. These test, then, can help an athlete avoid unnecessary periods of enforced rest. Whereas, a positive MRI can provide strong, visual reinforcement to help the athlete understand the need for often unwanted periods of enforced rest. Lastly, an MRI can be used, if necessary, to monitor progress and allow timely return to sport (early, but not too early, that is). Navicular stress fracture especially benefits from the sensitivity of MRI for timely diagnosis.

Plain x-rays will identify a Jones' fracture if it has progressed beyond a stress reaction (Figure 1). The fracture itself occurs at the metadiaphyseal area where the more flexible bone at the base of the 5th metatarsal meets the more rigid bone of the shaft of the metatarsal. The fracture is different from an avulsion fracture affecting the tip of the 5th metatarsal base.

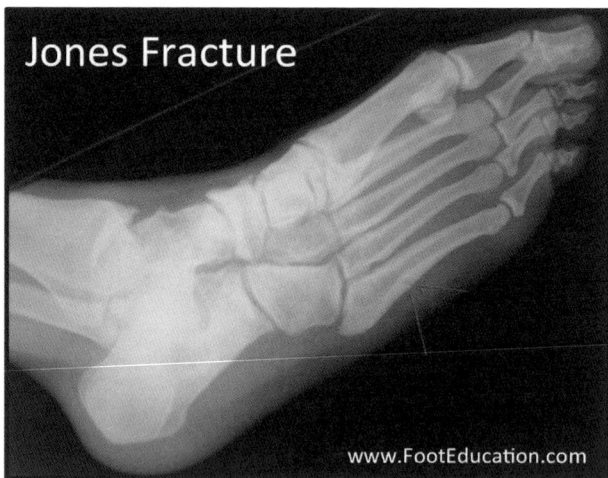

Figure 1: X-ray of Jones Fracture of the 5th Metatarsal

Routine x-rays of the foot can be very helpful in distinguishing a stress fracture of the sesamoid from a bipartite sesamoid. The distinction is that the bone fragments of a bipartite sesamoid have a clearly identified smooth margin, whereas a traumatic fracture has ragged edges. An x-ray of the contralateral foot can also be helpful given that the majority of bipartite sesamoids are bilateral. In some patients, an MRI or CT scan may be required to differentiate a bipartite sesamoid from a sesamoid stress fracture.

EPIDEMIOLOGY

Stress fractures are common and affect people of all ages. They are more likely to occur in females than in males, especially among females with the female athlete triad of amenorrhea, disordered eating, and osteoporosis. The estimated incidence in athletes and military recruits is 5-30%, depending on the sport and other risk factors. It is estimated that among people who run regularly for exercise, more than half will sustain an overuse injury that keeps them from running for 1 week. Stress fractures are among the more common injuries in recreational athletes. Stress fractures do not occur as often in the non-active population unless there is an underlying pathology that causes bone weakness or a sudden increase in activity level.

DIFFERENTIAL DIAGNOSIS

The main alternative diagnoses for stress fractures of the foot are trauma (including bone contusions) and tendinitis.

RED FLAGS

Stress fractures in a female athlete might be part of the Female Athletic Triad: namely, disordered eating, amenorrhea, and osteoporosis. Disordered eating (which may be manifest as compulsive exercising, as an indirect means of purging) leads to decreased body fat. Fat is a precursor of estrogen, therefore the level of this hormone is often much lower in emaciated women. Low levels of estrogen may lead to irregular menses and excessive bone resorption, as may be seen with osteoporosis. A poor diet also leads to inadequate bone maintenance owing to inadequate calcium and vitamin D intake as well.

TREATMENT OPTIONS AND OUTCOMES

Most stress fractures respond to rest. After all, stress fractures are overuse injuries, and rest (which may be thought of as "under-use") removes the harmful cause. For a stress fracture of the foot, immobilization and decreased weight-bearing which can be accomplished with crutches and a CAM walker boot may be helpful. For early injuries, cessation of the offending activity may be sufficient, often coupled with more supportive shoewear. For more involved stress fractures casting and non-weight-bearing may be necessary. Once healing has occurred, a gradual return to activity in a stiff-soled shoe is advised.

Certain stress fractures may benefit from surgery to aid in healing or prevent non-healing (i.e., non-union) or re-fracture. These "high risk" stress fractures include the Jones' fracture of the 5th metatarsal, navicular stress fractures, and those in other locations that have recurred despite adequate rest.

Surgery for a Jones' fracture stabilizes the fracture site by placing a screw through the canal of the bone (Figure 2). The screw itself resists deforming forces and the drilling needed to place it potentially stimulates blood flow to help healing. A patient that has a non-union of the Jones' fracture or a recurrent fracture after it had appeared to have healed, such as those with a significantly high arch, may need more involved reconstructive foot surgery to realign the foot and offload the fifth metatarsal more permanently.

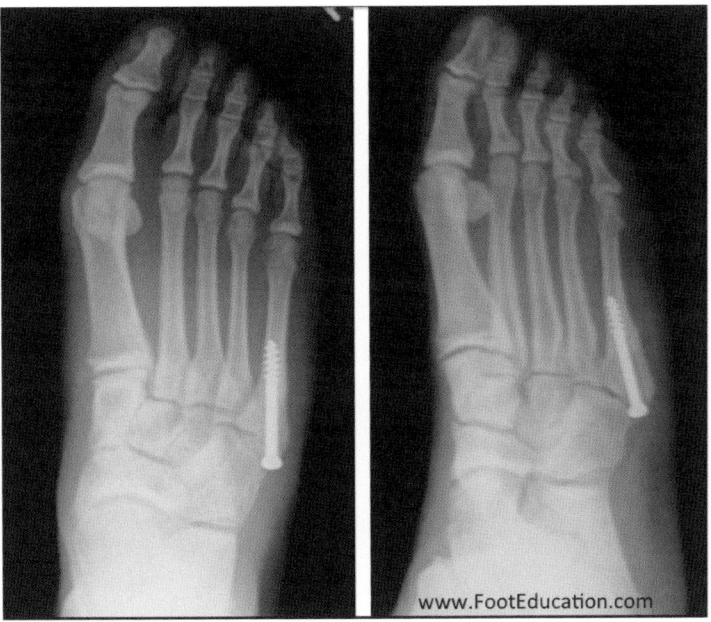

Figure 2: Screw Stabilization of a Jones Fracture

Navicular stress fractures can also be difficult to treat due to the relative lack of blood supply to the navicular. Nonetheless, treating non-displaced navicular stress fractures with casting and prolonged non-weight-bearing has been reported to be successful in 90% of cases if patients are compliant. Despite the lack of supportive evidence of efficacy, some doctors may also recommend use of a bone stimulating device which may employ electrical and electromagnetic stimulation, ultrasound, to extracorporeal shock waves to possibly encourage bone formation and growth. Early surgery may be recommended for some patients even without an initial period of non-operative treatment if there is any sign of fracture displacement, the period of needed immobilization is unacceptably long, or because the consequences of displacement may be too high. Surgery may be associated with a faster return to sports, and may include drilling across the fracture, placement of one or more screws, and possibly the addition of bone graft to improve healing.

Sesamoid stress fractures may be treated with an orthotic with a recess under the base of the first metatarsal head to transfer forces away from the sesamoids. This is combined with a cushioned insole and a stiff soled shoe with a rocker bottom contour to allow for a smoother dispersion of the force away from the base of the great toe. If this does not lead to symptom resolution, more aggressive immobilization and non-weight-bearing may be needed. The results of surgical treatment are unpredictable and thus surgery, in the form of repairing the fracture or removing part or all of the sesamoid bone, is often a treatment of last resort.

RISK FACTORS AND PREVENTION

Risk factors for stress fractures include intrinsic mechanical factors (e.g. decreased bone density, foot structure), nutritional factors, hormonal factors, physical training, and extrinsic mechanical factors (e.g. footwear, running surface). Patient's with metabolic bone diseases such as osteoporosis, osteomalacia, osteogenesis imperfecta, Paget's disease, and fibrous dysplasia are at a higher risk for stress fractures (insufficiency fractures).

Preventative measures to prevent stress fractures include gradually increasing training intensity, eating a diet with adequate amounts of calcium and vitamin D, and wearing the proper footwear for the desired activity as well as replacing footwear at appropriate intervals. For example, female military recruits given calcium and vitamin D supplements have been shown to be less likely to sustain a stress fracture than recruits that did not take supplements (PMID: 18433305). Runners may be able to prolong the longevity of their running shoes by considering them to be sports equipment using them specifically for running -and not for routine daily activities.

KEY TERMS

Stress fracture; Bone remodeling; osteoporosis; female athlete triad; Jones' fracture; navicular stress fracture; sesamoid stress fracture, calcium; vitamin D; amenorrhea; insufficiency fracture, fatigue fractures,

SKILLS

Bedside skills for the diagnosis stress fractures include the ability to take a detailed but focused history and perform a thorough musculoskeletal examination.

Printed in Great Britain
by Amazon